Essentials in Ophthalmology

Series Editor
Arun D. Singh

For further volumes:
http://www.springer.com/series/5332

Elizabeth P. Rakoczy

Editor

Arun D. Singh

Series Editor

Gene- and Cell-Based Treatment Strategies for the Eye

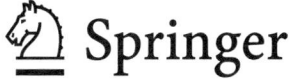 Springer

Editor
Elizabeth P. Rakoczy
Department of Molecular Ophthalmology
Centre for Ophthalmology and Visual Sciences
The University of Western Australia
Crawley
Western Australia
Australia

Series Editor
Arun D. Singh
Department of Ophthalmic Oncology
Cole Eye Institute
Cleveland Clinic
Cleveland, Ohio
USA

ISSN 1612-3212
ISBN 978-3-662-52329-2   ISBN 978-3-662-45188-5   (eBook)
DOI 10.1007/978-3-662-45188-5
Springer Heidelberg New York Dordrecht London

Preface

This book tells the great story of how the treatment of eye disease might change in the near future. The reader is explained how gene and cell therapies work and the difficulties scientists face in developing new technologies (experimental details, funding, approvals, ownership). The leaders of the field give a rare insight into the development of treatments for Leber's congenital amaurosis, choroideraemia, retintis pigmentosa, and macular degenerations that are expected to become part of the ophthalmologist's arsenal in the near future.

Crawley, WA, Australia   Elizabeth P. Rakoczy

Contents

Gene Therapy and Stem Cell Therapy: Overview

Aaron L. Magno, Samuel McLenachan,
and Elizabeth P. Rakoczy

1.1 Gene Therapy

In popular culture mutation has several meanings, but in this chapter mutation is used to refer to a nonlethal genetic change that is associated with a disease. Gene mutations can occur in a person in two ways: they can be inherited from a parent or acquired during a person's lifetime. Mutations that are passed from parent to child are called hereditary mutations. These types of mutations are present throughout a person's life in virtually every cell in the body including the germ cells, the sperm, and the egg; thus, they are passed on from one generation to the next. In contrast, mutations that occur in the building blocks of the body such as muscle, nerve, bone, blood, and gland cells – called somatic cells – are not inherited.

Why do mutations cause disease? The mutations in DNA can produce harmful proteins or negatively influence protein production in many ways. There are a wide range of mutations caused by change in a single or multiple nucleotides – missense, nonsense, insertion, frameshift, repeat expansion, and deletion mutations – that result in the insertion of an incorrect amino acid, shortening of the protein, change in reading the genetic code, or multiplication/deletion of certain amino acid sequences. Many disorders are caused by a mutation in a single gene. Approximately 4,000 disease-causing mutations in a variety of genes have already been identified, and for these the case-cause relationship between the mutation and a disease has been confirmed (McCarthy 2000). Depending on the location of the single base mutation in the genetic code and the change inflicted by it, the disease can be inherited in different ways. The inheritance pattern can be *dominant*, each affected individual has one affected parent and each child has a 50 % chance of inheriting the disease; *recessive*, an affected individual has unaffected parents who carry one copy of the mutated gene and each child has a 25 % chance of inheriting the disease; *X-linked dominant*, a mutation is carried on the X-chromosome by either parent, no male to male transmission; *X-linked recessive*, a mutation is carried on the X-chromosome by either parent and the majority of the offspring affected are male; *codominant*, two alleles are inherited together from different parents producing slightly different protein products and each child has a 25 % chance of inheriting the condition; and *mitochondrial*, a mutation

A.L. Magno, PhD
Department of Molecular Ophthalmology,
Lions Eye Institute, Perth, WA, Australia
e-mail: aaron.magno@lei.org.au

S. McLenachan, BSc(Hons), PhD
Department of Ocular Tissue Engineering,
Lions Eye Institute, Nedlands, WA, Australia
e-mail: smclenachan@lei.org.au

E.P. Rakoczy, PhD (✉)
Department of Molecular Ophthalmology, Centre for
Ophthalmology and Visual Sciences, The University
of Western Australia, Crawley, WA, Australia
e-mail: elizabeth.rakoczy@uwa.edu.au

E.P. Rakoczy (ed.), *Gene- and Cell-Based Treatment Strategies for the Eye*, Essentials in Ophthalmology,
DOI 10.1007/978-3-662-45188-5_1, © Springer-Verlag Berlin Heidelberg 2015

in the mitochondrial DNA, it can only be inherited from the mother, 100 % inheritance.

Diseases caused by many contributing factors are called complex or multifactorial disorders. Many common medical problems such as macular degeneration, heart disease, diabetes, and obesity do not have a single genetic cause but might be associated with changes in multiple genes with lifestyle and with environmental factors. Although complex disorders often cluster in families, they do not have a clear pattern of inheritance.

1.1.1 The Problem

The treatment of genetic disorders has proven to be difficult, and the majority of these conditions to date remain untreatable. Recently, the introduction of a new class of pharmaceuticals, called biopharmaceuticals, has offered some hope. Traditional pharmaceuticals interfere with a biological function by modifying the biological pathways. They are usually small synthetic molecules although there are examples that are produced by living organisms, like antibiotics. Biopharmaceuticals are active gene products or proteins that are produced by recombinant organisms. Functionally they have the potential of treating the underlying cause of a disease or correcting a genetic mutation. When a treatment uses a biopharmaceutical that can modify the genetic makeup of human cells with the introduction of a DNA code, it is called gene therapy.

1.1.2 The Solution

Gene therapy initially targeted diseases caused by the lack of a gene product due to a genetic mutation (Wolff and Lederberg 1994). However, with the development of technology, the definition of gene therapy has widened, and nowadays it refers to recombinant virus-delivered genes, nonviral-delivered genes, and gene-modifying technologies like antisense and RNAi technologies and targeted mutations.

Gene therapy aims to:
- Replace a mutated gene that causes disease with a healthy copy of the gene (Acland et al. 2001)

- Inactivate, or "knock out," a mutated gene that is functioning improperly (Farrar et al. 2012)
- Introduce a new gene into the body to help fight a disease (Lai et al. 2002)

One of the biggest barriers to the efficacy of gene therapy is the cell wall. Each cell, normal or diseased, is a small universe that fearlessly guards its barriers to maintain its own unique characteristics. Thus, for a successful gene therapy, a special carrier molecule, called a vector, must be used to penetrate the cell wall and force the cellular machinery to produce the therapeutic gene product.

Viruses have evolved a way of penetrating the cell wall, encapsulating and delivering their genes to human cells, albeit in a pathogenic manner. With the development of recombinant technologies, the viral genome can now be manipulated. The manipulation of the viral genome removes the disease-causing and replication genes but retains the genes useful for a vector (Vannucci et al. 2013). The space created by the removal of the disease-causing and replication genes is then used for the insertion of the therapeutic gene or transgene. Thus, recombinant viruses become carriers of the piece of human DNA that codes for the therapeutic gene. At present recombinant viruses are the most effective performing the double tasks of penetrating the cell wall and converting a mammalian cell to become a source of the therapeutic gene product. It is important to note that due to their genetic modifications, none of the recombinant viruses used as vectors can multiply.

The first step of recombinant virus-mediated gene delivery is the transduction of the target cells with the recombinant viral vector. The vector then unloads the genetic material into the cells that after a short delay start producing the therapeutic protein thus restoring normal function of the target cell.

Different types of viruses can be used as gene therapy vectors: retroviruses, lentiviruses, adenoviruses, herpes viruses, and adeno-associated viruses. In terms of ophthalmic applications, adeno-associated viruses have been extremely successful, and the rest of this chapter will concentrate on their description.

Adeno-associated viruses (AAV) are a class of small defective parvoviruses (Atchison et al. 1965; Hoggan et al. 1966). They are ubiquitous

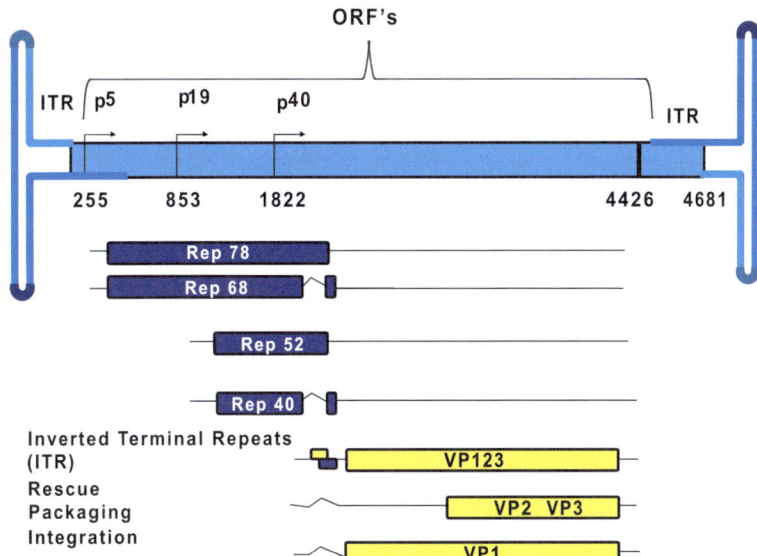

Fig. 1.1 Deriving recombinant adeno-associated virus (rAAV2) from its wild type. By the deletion of the ORFs, space is generated where a variety of transgenes can be introduced

in humans and appear to be nonpathogenic. The single-stranded DNA genome has two open reading frames which are flanked by two identical 145-base long inverted terminal repeats (ITR) (Fig. 1.1). AAVs have a wide host range and a stable virion.

AAV vectors or recombinant AAVs (rAAV) can transduce the muscle, liver, brain, retina, and lungs, but due to the fact that they are single-stranded DNAs, they require several weeks to reach optimal expression. The efficiency of rAAV transduction is dependent on the efficiency at each step of rAAV infection: binding, entry, viral trafficking, nuclear entry, uncoating, and second-strand synthesis (McCarty et al. 2004). Over 100 AAV serotypes or variants have been identified (Wu et al. 2006). These variants show slightly different characteristics of transduction efficiency and cell-type specificity. The most commonly used serotype for gene therapy is recombinant AAV2 (rAAV2) (Coura Rdos and Nardi 2007). rAAV2 contains only the two terminal repeats necessary for packaging, and all other viral coding sequences have been removed to make space for the transgene. The advantages of rAAV2 gene delivery are that it is nonpathogenic, has a wide host range, and does not require replicating cells. In addition due to the fact that rAAV vectors are capable of lytic infection in the presence of adenovirus, their large-scale production

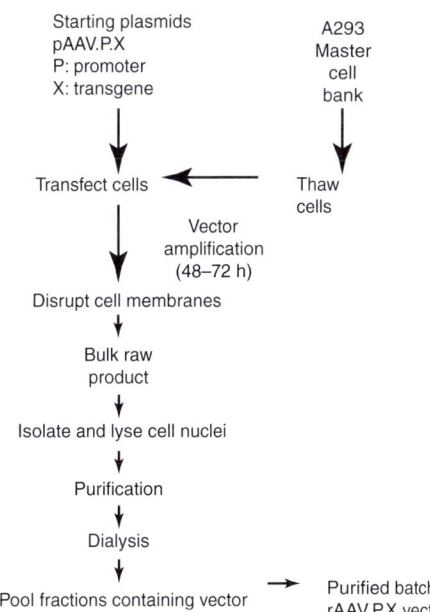

Fig. 1.2 rAAV production flowchart

is relatively easy compared to other recombinant viruses (Kotin 2011). With some variation all rAAV viruses presented in this book used similar manufacturing processes (Fig. 1.2).

The eye is an excellent target for gene therapy as it is a small organ that creates a confined space for the delivery, the retina-brain barrier limits the distribution of the rAAV into other organs, and its immune-privileged nature limits classical immune response. Via injections, a relatively easy, precise, and well-controlled delivery is available. Gene therapy in the eye requires small amounts of rAAV that have a huge impact on function, and there is a clearly defined and detectable end point. For the retina, the genome of rAAV2 has been widely used in research and has been thoroughly characterized (Rakoczy et al. 1999). rAAV2 has been the choice of vector for several of the clinical trials in this book.

1.1.3 Ethical Considerations

Initially, the new recombinant technologies made many people feel uncomfortable with what they called "the potential ability of scientist to change what it means to be a human." As a response scientists from around the world announced a voluntary moratorium on germline modification of human cells (i.e., modification of the genetic code in the sperm or in the egg), and some countries (Australia, New Zealand, the Netherlands, Canada, Germany, Switzerland) banned such research as they argued that the risks of injury to future generations outweighed the potential benefits. At the same time non-inherited, somatic gene therapy research and clinical trials were endorsed around the world with the caveat that special bodies had to oversee the clinical approval process of gene therapy products.

Nowadays somatic cell gene therapies are considered the extension of conventional therapies. It is widespread with more than 1,700 clinical trials conducted around the world. These trials demonstrated that somatic gene transfer or recombinant technologies did not represent a greater risk than other new therapeutics, and recently the American Society of Gene & Cell Therapy (ASGCT) called for an independent review of the clinical trial approval process and the activities of the National Institute of Health (NIH) Recombinant DNA Advisory Committee (RAC).

Dr. Xandra Breakefield president of ASGCT: The review and regulatory process already in place for these other investigational therapies do not include any equivalent to the RAC review for gene transfer technologies and appear to be more than adequate to assess both the unexpected off target toxicities or expected but severe side effects of many small molecule therapeutics and biologics, such as monoclonal antibodies or human recombinant proteins with potent systemic effects. Based on 20 years of safety data, it appears that it is long past time to bring the promise of gene transfer therapeutics out of its unique special status and into the mainstream of standard regulatory review that applies to the entire rest of the field of novel human therapeutics development.

Of course, gene therapy clinical trials will continue to fulfill the requirements of an ethical conduct: weighing potential harms and benefits, establishment of procedural fairness in selection of patients for research, assurance that consent to experimental treatments is informed and voluntary, and protection of privacy and confidentiality of medical information.

In 2012, Glybera, used for a rare genetic condition of lipoprotein lipase deficiency, became the first gene therapy treatment to be approved for clinical use in either Europe or the United States after its endorsement by the European Commission (Bryant et al. 2013).

1.2 Stem Cell Therapy

In contemporary biology, the phrase "stem cell" is used to describe a wide range of different precursor cell types, indicated by a variety of qualifying terms including "embryonic" and "adult" stem cells, "pluripotent" and "multipotent" stem cells, as well as tissue-specific varieties, such as neural and hematopoietic stem cells. In any of these contexts, the stem cell is a common precursor cell with an ability to self-renew for extended periods and give rise to more differentiated progeny. Stem cells are generally considered to possess "unlimited proliferation potential" and utilize a variety of mechanisms to protect the integrity of their genome and ensure their progeny inherit high-fidelity genetic information, including anaerobic metabolisms, long cell cycles, and increased expression of DNA repair and antioxidant proteins.

During development, only the zygote is considered totipotent, meaning it is capable of giving rise to all the different cell types of the organism. By the blastocyst stage, the totipotent cell has split into two new groups of stem cells, the tropho-blasts, which generate the placental tissues, and the inner cell mass comprised of pluripotent embryonic stem (ES) cells. ES cells are considered pluripotent, which means they can give rise to all the somatic cells of an organism, excluding the placental tissues. ES cells quickly disappear from the embryo, giving rise to the primordial germ layers of the ectoderm, mesoderm, and endoderm.

Following development stem cells are maintained in specialized niches in the adult. Stem cells are present in many adult tissues and organs, where they play important roles in replenishing cells lost during normal functioning (such as the shedding of keratinocytes from skin) or supplying progenitor cells for regenerative responses after injury.

1.2.1 Stem Cell Therapy

In principle, stem cell therapies (SCTs) aim to utilize the developmental potentials of stem cells to promote cellular regeneration and restore function to damaged or diseased tissues. One approach to this problem involves using growth factors to stimulate the proliferation of endogenous stem cells. This approach has shown great potential in the reactivation of stem cells in the mammalian spinal cord after injury. Exposure to basic fibroblast growth factor (FGF2) was shown to cause astrocytes in the injured mouse spinal cord to adopt a radial glial phenotype, bridging the lesion site and providing a scaffold for neuronal regeneration (Goldshmit et al. 2014).

The recruitment of endogenous stem cell populations for tissue regeneration may not be possible when a large numbers of cells have been lost or when dealing with aged stem cell pools. Similarly, patients suffering genetic diseases may require donor cells from other individuals or a combined gene therapy-cell therapy approach in which cells are removed and genetically modified before being delivered back to the patient. To address these clinical needs, great efforts have been made toward the isolation and culture of adult stem cells for SCTs.

Adult stem cells can be isolated from various accessible tissues throughout the human body.

Neural stem cells can be obtained from biopsies of the olfactory epithelium. Alternately, Schwann cells of the peripheral nerves and neural crest-derived stem cells present in the hair follicle have been shown to possess neural stem cell potential. In most stratified epithelia, epithelial stem cells are dispersed in the basal layers, where they give rise to dividing progenitors that terminally differentiate as they rise to the surface. In the lining of the gut and in the corneoscleral limbus of the eye, epithelial stem cells are located in crypts or palisades. The mesoderm and neural crest collectively give rise to numerous mesenchymal stem cell (MSC) populations in the adult, including the bone marrow and adipose stem cells as well as limbal mesenchymal stem cells, which are scattered throughout the limbal and corneal stroma.

Since the early successes of bone marrow transplant (BMT) therapies, much attention has been placed on the potential for MSC in the treatment of a number of diseases. MSC are defined by their ability expanded over many passages in culture and differentiated into osteoblasts, adipose cells, and chondrocytes. However, in addition to multipotency MSC have been shown to possess immunomodulatory and trophic support properties that may contribute to their therapeutic efficacy (Bray et al. 2014).

1.2.2 Limbal Stem Cell Therapy

Since the development of BMT in the 1960s, progress in clinical cell therapies has been slow, with the first successful limbal epithelial transplant reported in 1989, marking the beginning of limbal stem cell therapy (LSCT). The corneal epithelium is constantly replenished with new cells originating from limbal epithelial stem cells (LESCs), located at the corneoscleral junction. LESCs are dispersed in a specialized niche, known as limbal palisades or crypts.

Damage to the limbal niche can lead to limbal stem cell deficiency, a painful and debilitating condition resulting in the destabilization and loss of corneal epithelium and the ingrowth of the vascular conjunctival epithelium over the cornea and a loss of vision in the affected eye. Transplantation of healthy limbal tissue (Kenyon and Tseng 1989) or limbal cell cultures containing >3 % LESCs (Pellegrini et al. 1997; Rama et al. 2010) was found to restore the integrity and transparency of the corneal surface.

Although still under development, limbal stem cell transplantation has been successfully employed in numerous clinical trials (Harkin et al. 2013). However, Daya's demonstration that no donor cell DNA could be detected on the corneal surface 9 months after transplantation (Daya et al. 2005) raises questions about the therapeutic mechanism of this "stem cell therapy," since replacement of LESCs does not seem to occur. For the corneal surface to contain only host DNA, the LESC pool must be recruited from spared host LESCs, which may occur after remodeling of the limbal niche in response to the transplanted cells.

1.2.3 Pluripotent Stem Cells

Although the United Nations Educational, Scientific and Cultural Organization's (UNESCO) 1997 Universal Declaration on the Human Genome and Human Rights states that reproductive cloning shall not be permitted as it is contrary to human dignity, a later report from the UNESCO international bioethics committee in 2001 acknowledged human ES cell research is of considerable interest and recommended governments debate the issue and decide for themselves. While a number of countries, such as the United States and Australia, responded by placing restrictions on the creation of new ES cell lines, ES cell research has continued using previously established lines as well as lines generated in countries with fewer restrictions.

To date, ES-derived cells have been used in two Phase I clinical trials. The first, announced by Geron in 2009, was for the treatment of spinal cord injury; however, the trial was discontinued due to economic restraints and the results never published. The second, in which ES cell-derived retinal pigment epithelial cells were transplanted into two patients with macular degeneration, is discussed in Chap. 4 (Schwartz et al. 2012).

In 2006, Shinya Yamanaka and Kazutoshi Takahashi reported the reprogramming of mouse fibroblasts to a pluripotent state, using retroviruses to deliver genes encoding four transcription factors (Takahashi and Yamanaka 2006). Forced expression of the Yamanaka factors, OCT4, SOX2, KLF4, and C-MYC was found to induce a similar phenotype to mouse ES cells through induction and stabilization of a core network of transcription factors, including OCT4, SOX2, and NANOG that regulate the gene expression profile required for the pluripotent state. Like embryonic carcinoma cells, "induced pluripotent stem (iPS) cells" were shown to contribute to chimerism after blastocyst injection and form teratomas with trilineage differentiation potential in mice. Human iPS cells were independently generated by three groups in the year following Yamanaka's paper (Takahashi et al. 2007; Yu et al. 2007; Park et al. 2008) and were heralded with the promise of accessible pluripotent cultures derived from patients. This advance offers a significant advantage over stem cell therapies being developed using human ES cells in that the donor cells can be genetically matched to the patient, avoiding the potential need for immunosuppression after transplantation. However, the integrity of human iPS cells and their safety for use in clinical applications remain controversial. Evidence of incomplete reprogramming, persistence of epigenetic heritage (Ruiz et al. 2012), as well as mutation rates in iPS cells more similar to differentiated cells than ES cells (Kruta et al. 2014) has been demonstrated, suggesting further refinement of iPS cell induction and quality control measures may be required before clinical implementation can be made safe (McLenachan et al. 2012; Palomo et al. 2014).

1.2.4 Future of Stem Cell Therapies

The clinical success stories of BMT and LSCT represent the first steps on the road to stem cell therapies, providing useful lessons that may be applied to the development of therapies using other types of stem cells and for different target tissues. However, the field of SCT remains in its developmental stages. This is likely in part due to the multidisciplinary nature of stem cell therapies, which brings together diverse aspects of cellular, molecular, and developmental biology, physiology, immunology, and surgery as well as materials engineering and other disciplines, all of which must attain sufficient maturity for the successful realization of tissue engineering and cellular replacement strategies. The discoveries of the human genome sequence, adult and pluripotent stem cells, as well as cellular reprogramming techniques represent key components in the expanding toolbox of medical research. As the challenges of integrating these new discoveries into the development of gene and stem cell therapies are met, exciting new approaches to human diseases are becoming possible.

Compliance with Ethical Requirements Elizabeth Rakoczy, Samuel McLenachan, and Aaron Magno declare that they have no conflict of interest.

No animal or human studies were carried out by the authors of this chapter.

References

Acland GM, Aguirre GD, Ray J, Zhang Q, Aleman TS, Cideciyan AV et al (2001) Gene therapy restores vision in a canine model of childhood blindness. Nat Genet 28:92–95

Atchison RW, Casto BC, Hammon WM (1965) Adenovirus-associated defective virus particles. Science 149:754–756

Bray LJ, Heazlewood CF, Munster DJ, Hutmacher DW, Atkinson K, Harkin DG (2014) Immunosuppressive properties of mesenchymal stromal cell cultures derived from the limbus of human and rabbit corneas. Cytotherapy 16:64–73

Bryant LM, Christopher DM, Giles AR, Hinderer C, Rodriguez JL, Smith JB et al (2013) Lessons learned from the clinical development and market authorization of Glybera. Hum Gene Ther Clin Dev 24:55–64

Coura Rdos S, Nardi NB (2007) The state of the art of adeno-associated virus-based vectors in gene therapy. Virol J 4:99

Daya SM, Watson A, Sharpe JR, Giledi O, Rowe A, Martin R et al (2005) Outcomes and DNA analysis of ex vivo expanded stem cell allograft for ocular surface reconstruction. Ophthalmology 112:470–477

Farrar GJ, Millington-Ward S, Chadderton N, Humphries P, Kenna PF (2012) Gene-based therapies for dominantly inherited retinopathies. Gene Ther 19:137–144

Goldshmit Y, Frisca F, Pinto AR, Pebay A, Tang JK, Siegel AL et al (2014) Fgf2 improves functional recovery-decreasing gliosis and increasing radial glia and neural progenitor cells after spinal cord injury. Brain Behav 4:187–200

Harkin DG, Apel AJ, Di Girolamo N, Watson S, Brown K, Daniell MD et al (2013) Current status and future prospects for cultured limbal tissue transplants in Australia and New Zealand. Clin Experiment Ophthalmol 41:272–281

Hoggan MD, Blacklow NR, Rowe WP (1966) Studies of small DNA viruses found in various adenovirus preparations: physical, biological, and immunological characteristics. Proc Natl Acad Sci U S A 55:1467–1474

Kenyon KR, Tseng SC (1989) Limbal autograft transplantation for ocular surface disorders. Ophthalmology 96:709–722; discussion 22–23

Kotin RM (2011) Large-scale recombinant adeno-associated virus production. Hum Mol Genet 20:R2–R6

Kruta M, Seneklova M, Raska J, Salykin A, Zerzankova L, Pesl M et al (2014) Mutation frequency dynamics in HPRT locus in culture adapted human embryonic stem cells and induced pluripotent stem cells correspond to their differentiated counterparts. Stem Cells Dev 23:2443–2454

Lai YK, Shen WY, Brankov M, Lai CM, Constable IJ, Rakoczy PE (2002) Potential long-term inhibition of ocular neovascularisation by recombinant adeno-associated virus-mediated secretion gene therapy. Gene Ther 9:804–813

McCarthy A (2000) Pharmacogenetics: implications for drug development, patients and society. N Genet Soc 19:135–143

McCarty DM, Young SM Jr, Samulski RJ (2004) Integration of adeno-associated virus (AAV) and recombinant AAV vectors. Annu Rev Genet 38:819–845

McLenachan S, Menchon C, Raya A, Consiglio A, Edel MJ (2012) Cyclin A1 is essential for setting the pluripotent state and reducing tumorigenicity of induced pluripotent stem cells. Stem Cells Dev 21:2891–2899

Palomo AB, McLenachan S, Osete JR, Menchon C, Barrot C, Chen F et al (2014) Plant hormones increase efficiency of reprogramming mouse somatic cells to induced pluripotent stem cells and reduce tumorigenicity. Stem Cells Dev 23:586–593

Park IH, Zhao R, West JA, Yabuuchi A, Huo H, Ince TA et al (2008) Reprogramming of human somatic cells to pluripotency with defined factors. Nature 451:141–146

Pellegrini G, Traverso CE, Franzi AT, Zingirian M, Cancedda R, De Luca M (1997) Long-term restoration of damaged corneal surfaces with autologous cultivated corneal epithelium. Lancet 349:990–993

Rakoczy PE, Shen W-Y, Lai M, Rolling F, Constable IJ (1999) Development of gene therapy-based strategies for the treatment of eye diseases. Drug Dev Res 46:277–285

Rama P, Matuska S, Paganoni G, Spinelli A, De Luca M, Pellegrini G (2010) Limbal stem-cell therapy and long-term corneal regeneration. N Engl J Med 363:147–155

Ruiz S, Diep D, Gore A, Panopoulos AD, Montserrat N, Plongthongkum N et al (2012) Identification of a specific reprogramming-associated epigenetic signature in human induced pluripotent stem cells. Proc Natl Acad Sci 109:16196–16201

Schwartz SD, Hubschman JP, Heilwell G, Franco-Cardenas V, Pan CK, Ostrick RM et al (2012) Embryonic stem cell trials for macular degeneration: a preliminary report. Lancet 379:713–720

Takahashi K, Tanabe K, Ohnuki M, Narita M, Ichisaka T, Tomoda K et al (2007) Induction of pluripotent stem cells from adult human fibroblasts by defined factors. Cell 131:861–872

Takahashi K, Yamanaka S (2006) Induction of pluripotent stem cells from mouse embryonic and adult fibroblast cultures by defined factors. Cell 126: 663–676

Vannucci L, Lai M, Chiuppesi F, Ceccherini-Nelli L, Pistello M (2013) Viral vectors: a look back and ahead on gene transfer technology. New Microbiol 36:1–22

Wolff JA, Lederberg J (1994) An early history of gene transfer and therapy. Hum Gene Ther 5:469–480

Wu Z, Asokan A, Samulski RJ (2006) Adeno-associated virus serotypes: vector toolkit for human gene therapy. Mol Ther 14:316–327

Yu J, Vodyanik MA, Smuga-Otto K, Antosiewicz-Bourget J, Frane JL, Tian S et al (2007) Induced pluripotent stem cell lines derived from human somatic cells. Science 318:1917–1920

Gene Therapy for Leber's Congenital Amaurosis Due to *RPE65* Mutations

Jean Bennett

2.1   Description of the Disease

Leber's congenital amaurosis (LCA) refers to a group of hereditary, early-onset retinal degenerative conditions characterized by severe impairment in retinal and visual function. Diagnosis is usually made during the first few months of life in infants who present with severely impaired vision, abnormal eye movements (nystagmus), and abnormal electroretinograms (ERG) reflecting decreased retinal function. The (poor) vision that is present at birth progressively deteriorates through loss of photoreceptors, typically leading to total blindness by the third or fourth decade of life (Aleman et al. 2004; Lorenz et al. 2000; Simonelli et al. 2007; Perrault et al. 1999).

LCA is usually inherited as an autosomal recessive trait, and mutations in at least 18 different genes have been reported so far (RetNet 2014). At present, there are no approved treatments available for LCA.

This development program focuses on one form of LCA, *LCA2*, caused by mutations in the gene encoding the human retinal pigment epithelium 65 kDa protein, *hRPE65* (Morimura et al.

1998; Thompson et al. 2005). The *RPE65* gene encodes an enzyme (retinal pigment epithelium 65 kDa protein (RPE65)), produced by the retinal pigment epithelium (RPE), retinal isomerohydrolase. This enzyme is necessary for production of a vitamin A derivative, 11-cis retinal, which in turn is necessary for vision (Redmond et al. 1998). Without 11-cis retinal, rhodopsin cannot be formed, and light stimuli exposing the retina cannot be transformed to electrical signals (Redmond et al. 1998; Redmond and Hamel 2000). The biochemical blockade of the visual cycle resulting from *RPE65* deficiency causes a profound impairment in visual function and visual perception. Further, there is a slow degeneration of retinal photoreceptors which may result, in part, from toxicity due to buildup of the 11-cis retinal (retinoid ester) precursors in the RPE cells.

At present, there are no approved treatments available for LCA. The avenue that is being explored is gene augmentation therapy, whereby the wild-type version of the human *RPE65* cDNA is delivered to retinal pigment epithelium (RPE) cells, allowing these cells to then produce the RPE65 protein. The *hRPE65* cDNA is delivered through a one-time exposure to recombinant adeno-associated virus (AAV). LCA2 is an excellent candidate for a gene augmentation therapy approach: (i) molecular testing is available to identify individuals with mutation(s) in the *RPE65* gene; (ii) the route of administration is based on existing standard human retinal surgery techniques; (iii) small volumes of gene transfer

J. Bennett, MD, PhD
Department of Ophthalmology, F.M. Kirby Center for Molecular Ophthalmology, Center for Advanced Retinal and Ophthalmic Therapeutics, The Children's Hospital of Philadelphia, University of Pennsylvania, Perelman School of Medicine, Philadelphia, PA, USA
e-mail: jebennet@mail.med.upenn.edu

material can be delivered to the subretinal space thereby preferentially exposing the diseased cells; (iv) there is minimal systemic exposure to the gene transfer agent. This reduces the potential of systemic complications and thus of a toxic immune response (Acland et al. 2005; Bennicelli et al. 2008; Jacobson et al. 2006; Maguire et al. 2008, 2009; Hauswirth et al. 2008); (v) the relative immune-privilege enjoyed by the eye may facilitate prolonged expression; (vi) the target cells in the retina are terminally differentiated at birth, and therefore it is unlikely that the reagent would be diluted by cell division; (vii) proof of concept of gene augmentation therapy has been demonstrated in both large and small animal models using the human gene (Acland et al. 2001, 2005; Dejneka et al. 2004a; Narfstrom et al. 2001, 2003a, b, c; Bennicelli et al. 2008). Those studies documented rapid onset of improvement in retinal and visual function in a stable fashion with a high level of safety; (viii) improvement of retinal function has been reported for multiple subjects through AAV-mediated *RPE65* delivery in three separate Phase I clinical studies, and several other Phase I trials are in progress (Table 2.1) (Maguire et al. 2008, 2009; Hauswirth et al. 2008; Jacobson et al. 2012; Cideciyan et al. 2008, 2009a, b; Bainbridge et al. 2008; Banin et al. 2010). The early reports from the first three contemporaneous trials reveal a high degree of safety and demonstrate efficacy as judged by increase in light sensitivity, improved visual acuity and visual fields, improved pupillary light reflex and improved mobility (Maguire et al. 2008, 2009; Bainbridge et al. 2008; Hauswirth et al. 2008). Two of the trials have reported long-term results, and the results indicate that the initial gains in function have been maintained (Bennett et al. 2012; Simonelli et al. 2010; Jacobson et al. 2012; Cideciyan et al. 2013). The majority of the studies employed an AAV serotype 2 vector delivering the wild-type human *RPE65* cDNA subretinally to the RPE in one eye (Table 2.1), but the studies differed in terms of dose, inclusion criteria, type of promoter, location of injection, and outcome measures; (ix) there is also evidence of improvement in retinal function in a follow-on Phase I/II study, carried out at the Children's Hospital

of Philadelphia (CHOP) (Bennett et al. 2012). This study involved readministration of the vector to the contralateral eye of eligible individuals involved in the initial Phase I dose-escalation study (Table 2.1).

2.2 The Road to Gene Therapy for LCA

As technology developed allowing one to clone and manipulate DNA, and demonstration was made in animals that delivery of cloned genes into the germ line could alter the phenotype of the animals, the obvious next step was to test somatic gene delivery for the amelioration or even cure of disease. It took several decades, however, for all of the necessary tools/reagents to be assembled. The retina became an interesting target once the first two blindness-associated genes were identified, choroideremia (CHM), implicated in an X-linked retinal degenerative condition, and rhodopsin (RHO), most frequent cause of retinitis pigmentosa (RP) (Cremers et al. 1990; Nathans and Hogness 1984; Dryja et al. 1990; Humphries et al. 1990).

I had been aiming in the 1980s to develop gene transfer approaches for systemic diseases, but realized once the retinal genes were identified, that monogenic diseases of the retina were excellent targets. My first experiments with the retina aimed to develop safe and stable methods of retinal gene transfer. There were two parts to this problem: one surgical and one relating to gene transfer efficiency and stability. The surgical approaches were developed through work carried out with long-term collaborator, Albert M. Maguire, MD. Dr. Maguire, while a fellow in retina surgery, received a pilot grant from Fight for Sight; simultaneously, I received a career development award from the then "Retinitis Pigmentosa Foundation," currently Foundation Fighting Blindness (FFB). With the support of these patient-oriented organizations, we developed surgical methods in large and small animal models that could be extrapolated eventually to humans. These approaches initially used physicochemical methods to transfect the *LacZ*

Table 2.1 Details of vectors and clinical trials used evaluating gene augmentation therapy for LCA2. Details were obtained from the www.clinicaltrials.gov listing, media reports, and/or published results

Surgery site	Clinical trials.gov ID	PI	Phase	Initiation date	Name of vector	Source of vector	AAV capsid	Promoter	Poly (A)	Dose/Eye (vg)	Volume (µl)	# Subjects	Lowest baseline VA (LogMAR)	Additional
Moorefields (London, UK)	NCT00643747	R.R. Ali	I/II	2008	AAVAAG76 (rAAV2/2.hRPE65p.hRPE65)	TG	2	hRPE65; 1400 bp	bGH	≤1.00E11	≤1,000	9	1.52	Small detachment generated before injecting AAV
CHOP; Philadelphia, PA, USA	NCT00516477	A.M. Maguire	I/II	2008	AAV2-hRPE65v2	CCMT/CHOP	2	CBA	bGH	1.5E10-1.5E11	150-300	12	3.5a-0.96	Pluronic F-68 in Excipient
UGainesville, Gainesville, FL, USA	NCT00481546	S.G. Jacobson	I/II	2008	AAV2-CBSB-hRPE65	AGTC	2	CBA (short CMV)	SV40	5.96E10-1.788E11	150-450	15	1.96 (most were ~1.1)	Some received multiple injections
Hadassah-HUMC, Jerusalem, Israel	NCT00821340	E. Banin	I	2010	AAV2-CB-hRPE65	AGTC	2	CBA (long CMV)	SV40	1.19E11	300	NA	NA (≤0.4)	
OHSU; UMass, Portland, OR; Worcester, MA, USA	NCT00749957	J.T. Stout	I	2011	rAAV2-CB-hRPE65	AGTC	2	CBA (long CMV)	SV40	1.8E11 6E11	450	12	NA (≤0.48)	
Nantes U Hospital, Nantes, France	NCT01496040	M. Weber	I	2011	rAAV2/4.hRPE65	Genethon	4	NA	NA	NA	400-800	9	NA (<0.32)	
CHOP; Philadelphia, PA; UIowa, Iowa City, IA, USA	NCT00999609	A.M. Maguire, S.R. Russell	III	2012	AAV2-hRPE65v2	CHOP	2	CBA	bGH	1.50E11	300	24	NA (<0.48)	Pluronic F-68 in Excipient
CHOP; Philadelphia, PA, USA	NCT01208389	A.M. Maguire	I/II FO	2010	AAV2-hRPE65v2	CHOP	2	CBA	bGH	1.50E11	300	12	3.5a-0.45	Pluronic F-68 in Excipient

CBA chicken beta actin promoter with cytomegalovirus (CMV) enhancer, *CB* CBA promoter with long CMV enhancer, *CBSB* CBA promoter with short CMV enhancer, *TG* targeted genetics, *CCMT/CHOP* Center for Cellular and Molecular Therapeutics at the Children's Hospital of Philadelphia, *Moorefields* Moorefields Eye Hospital, *UGainesville* University of Gainesville Hospital, *Hadassah-HUMC* Hadassah-Hebrew University Medical Center, *Nantes* Nantes University Hospital, *OHSU* Oregon Hospital State University (Rojas-Burke 2011), *UMass* University of Massachusetts, Worcester, *UIowa* University of Iowa Hospital, *vg* vector genomes, *bGH* bovine growth hormone, *SV40* simian virus 40, *NA* not available

aVisual acuity was between hand motion and light perception and so was assigned LogMAR 3.5

reporter gene, which encodes histochemically detectable beta-galactosidase (β-Gal).

Simultaneously, other investigators had been developing recombinant adenovirus vectors, which transduce respiratory cells efficiently, and thus might have been useful for gene therapy studies of cystic fibrosis (CF). We used our newly developed surgical techniques to evaluate retinal somatic gene transfer using first-generation recombinant adenoviral vectors. Because little was known about the safety of Ad vectors, our studies were carried out using biohazard level 3 facilities – i.e., facilities with air locks, full body protective apparel, and sequestration of the animals. [Animal studies using recombinant Ad vectors are usually now carried out using level 2 facilities.] Subretinal injection of Ad.CMV.LacZ led to expression of high levels and early-onset (within 48 h) expression of the β-Gal reporter gene in RPE and Muller cells of adult mice and in photoreceptor precursor cells in neonatal mice (Bennett et al. 1994; Li et al. 1994). An Ad vector, in which the βPDE cDNA was exchanged for the β-Gal cDNA, and the retinal degeneration (rd) mouse model, was then used to demonstrate the first proof of concept of in vivo retinal gene therapy (Bennett et al. 1996). Because of its immunogenic potential, its inefficient transduction of mature photoreceptors, and the lack of stability of transgene expression, we and others began to search for alternative recombinant viral vectors. The first retinal studies with adeno-associated virus (AAV) demonstrated the advantages of AAV over adenovirus: efficient and stable transduction of retinal cells with a favorable immune profile; (Fig. 2.1; Ali et al. 1996; Bennett et al. 1997; Flannery et al. 1997). AAV serotype 2 (AAV2) was the first AAV serotype identified and thus the first to be studied. AAV is a nonpathogenic, single-stranded DNA genome-containing, helper virus-dependent member of the parvovirus family. AAV particles are small (~26 nm diameter) non-enveloped, icosahedral virions (Carter 1996). Jomary was the first to use AAV to demonstrate proof of concept of gene therapy in an animal model (the rd mouse model of RP) (Jomary et al. 1997).

From 2001 to 2005, I undertook countless discussions with small and large pharma to

determine whether there was corporate interest in supporting a potentially expensive Phase 1 gene therapy clinical trial for LCA2. Although there was great interest and the leaders were genuinely impressed with the proof-of-concept data, the fact that LCA2 is an ultra-orphan disease had a negative impact on decisions to support a study financially. The outlook changed, though, in July 2005, when Dr. Katherine High presented me/my team an invitation to carry out a clinical trial at CHOP. She had just established a Center for Cellular and Molecular Therapeutics (CCMT) at CHOP, complete with a GMP vector core and relevant expertise in regulatory affairs. She had recruited world-renowned experts in design of gene therapy clinical studies from a gene therapy company (Avigen) that had just folded. With the regulatory/vector expertise and financial backing secure, we were able to join forces and move forward to carry out LCA2 clinical studies without delay.

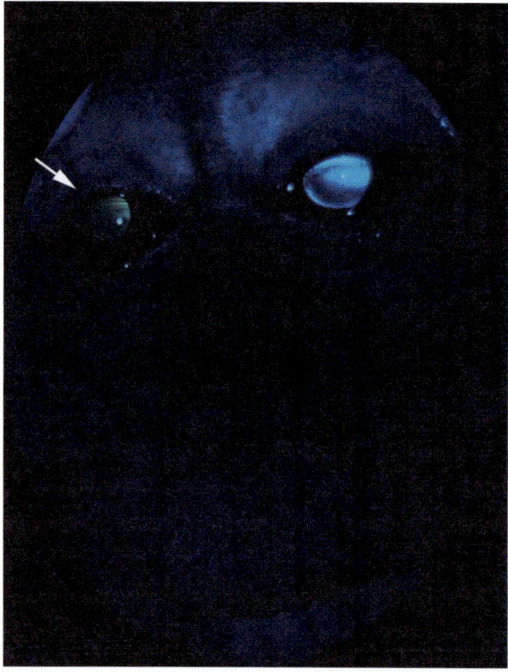

Fig. 2.1 Representative retinal transgene expression 3 months after subretinal delivery of 1E10 vector genomes (vg) AAV.CMV.GFP in a non-human primate (Vandenberghe et al. 2013). Green fluorescent protein (GFP) expressed by retinal cells make the retina glow green (*arrow*) after illumination with a blue light

2.3 Major Milestones in the Discovery

2.3.1 Identification of *RPE65*-Mediated Disease in Humans and Animal Models

Mutations in the *RPE65* gene were first identified as the cause of Leber's congenital amaurosis (LCA) in 1997. These included missense, point mutations, and rearrangements (Gu et al. 1997; Marlhens et al. 1997). This gene then became a candidate gene for the retinal disease found in Swedish Briard dogs that had previously been diagnosed with congenital stationary night blindness by Dr. K. Narfstrom et al. (1989). The Swedish Briard *RPE65* mutation, a 4 bp deletion causing a frameshift and a premature stop codon, was identified in the late 1990s (Aguirre et al. 1998; Veske et al. 1999). In the *RPE65−/−* dog, the mutation was found to cause retinal and visual dysfunction and RPE accumulation of lipid vacuoles. An appealing feature of this disease with respect to gene therapy was that the gene was expressed in RPE cells, which are very efficiently transduced by viral vectors, and that there was a slowly progressive retinal degeneration, thereby allowing a window of opportunity for gene therapy-based intervention. It thus became logical to consider testing the possibility of AAV-mediated rescue of LCA2 in the *RPE65* dog model. The dog model was available prior to the engineered mutant *Rpe65−/−* mouse (1998) (Redmond et al. 1998), and a spontaneous mutant *Rpe65−/−* ("rd12") mouse was (2005) (Pang et al. 2005).

2.3.2 Identification of the Delivery Vector

Although the first recombinant virus evaluated, adenovirus, efficiently transduces RPE and Muller cells and leads to both a rapid onset and high level of transgene expression, it quickly became apparent that this virus is highly immunogenic and that transduction results in only transient transgene expression (Maguire et al. 1995; Borras et al. 1996; Hoffman et al. 1997). The subsequent death in one human injected with Ad systemically in a study of gene therapy for ornithine transcarbamylase deficiency (Wade 1999) made this virus even less attractive. In 1996–1997, when several groups demonstrated efficient and stable transgene expression after delivery of recombinant AAV2 vectors to retina (see above), focus quickly shifted to this vector. AAV vectors do not carry any virus open reading frames and thus do not deliver any virus-specific proteins. This is an advantage (compared to adenovirus) as it limits the potential of development of a harmful immunogenic response to foreign antigens. Recombinant AAV vectors also target a more diverse set of cell types than other vectors and do not carry a high risk of insertional mutagenesis (since they rarely integrate) (Carter 1996). Once the AAV infects the cell, the DNA travels to and persists in episomal fashion in the nucleus of the target cells. Expression from the transgene cassette persists for the life of small animals (rodents) and was later shown to persist for significant periods of time (at least 11 years in dogs) after subretinal injection (Acland et al. 2005; Cideciyan et al. 2013) When using AAV to deliver the jellyfish-derived green fluorescent protein (GFP) reporter gene, one can visualize transgene expression in the retina long after injection (Fig. 2.1). A disadvantage of AAV vectors is that they have a relatively limited cargo capacity (4.8 kb); however, that is not a limitation for the *RPE65* cDNA. Thus, AAV2 rapidly became the vector of choice for retinal gene delivery for LCA2.

2.3.3 The Construct

The constructs used in the three original trials were similar in that they all used the *hRPE65* cDNA and AAV2; however, they (and the ensuing trials) differed in other variables (Table 2.1). [Only one of the more recent trials has used a different AAV capsid (AAV4).] The AAVs differed in details of the promoter/enhancer, presence of a Kozak sequence, and whether or not there was a stuffer sequence in the proviral plasmid (Fig. 2.2). The latter modification prevents reverse packaging from the

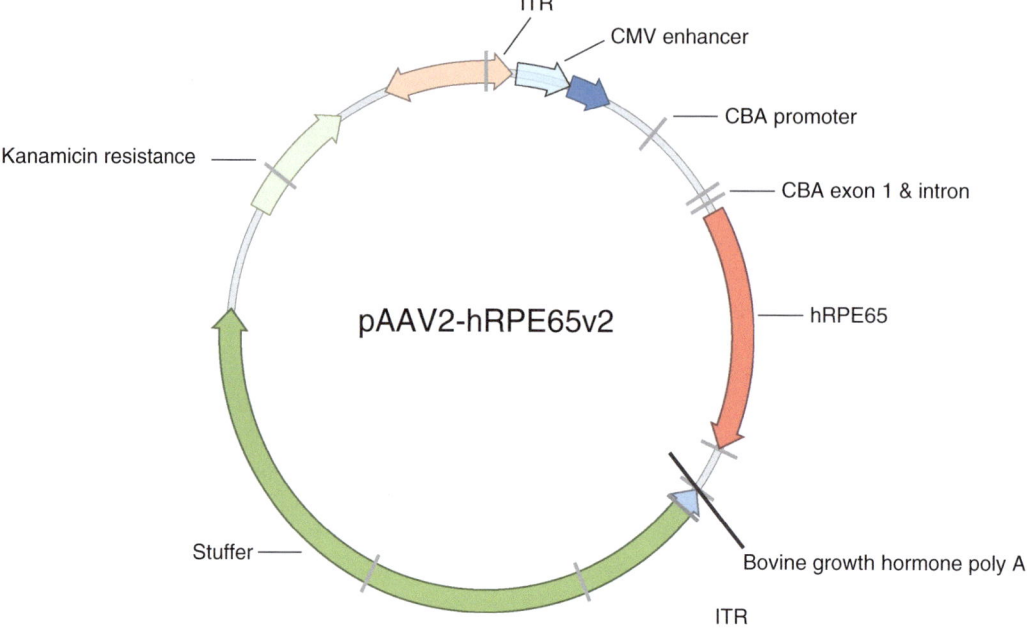

Fig. 2.2 Map of the proviral plasmid used to generate AAV2.hRPE65v2 by the team at the Children's Hospital of Philadelphia. The human RPE65 cDNA is driven by a chicken beta actin (CBA) promoter and a cytomegalovirus (CMV) enhancer, and there is a bovine growth hormone poly(A). Only the segment between the inverted terminal repeats (ITRs) is packaged in the virus. The proviral plasmid also contains a kanamycin resistance gene for selection and a noncoding stuffer sequence, used to prevent reverse packaging (Bennicelli et al. 2008). This minimizes the formation of empty capsids

AAV inverted terminal repeats (ITRs), possible when the size of the vector plasmid backbone is less than the packaging limit of AAV. Reverse packaging would result in empty vector (i.e., vector lacking the transgene cassette). This feature was thus thought to enhance safety while maximizing therapeutic effect. The AAV vector that we have used at CHOP, pAAV.CMV.CβA. hRPE65v2, contains a cytomegalovirus (CMV) immediate early enhancer, a chicken β-actin (CβA) promoter, the human *RPE65* cDNA (including intron and open reading frame), and a downstream bovine growth hormone poly A sequence (Fig. 2.2). This plasmid backbone has the following characteristics besides the stuffer sequence: (1) it contains a kanamycin resistance gene for selection and growth; (2) it contains a bacterial origin of replication; and (3) it contains inverted terminal repeats from AAV2. The excipient for the CHOP vector was

phosphate-buffed saline containing 0.001 % Pluronic F68. Pluronic F68 is a surfactant that prevents absorption of vector to inert surfaces (such as the insides of storage vessels and injection devices) and thus allows accurate dosing (Bennicelli et al. 2008). None of the other studies used surfactant in the excipient.

2.3.4   In Vitro Data

We first tested AAV.RPE65 vectors in vitro in primary canine RPE cell cultures using a canine cDNA (cloned by Jharna Ray) and demonstrated that the treated *RPE65−/−* cells were able to produce the wild-type RPE65 protein after infection (Acland et al. 2001). In vitro studies revealed no evidence of toxicity to the exposed cells and no signs of abnormal cell division or increased amounts of apoptotic cell death after transduction with AAV.RPE65. Later studies using a human RPE65 cDNA (cloned by Nadine Dejneka) and the additional modifications described in Table 2.1 showed similar results (Bennicelli, unpublished data). Importantly, the in vitro data demonstrated that transduction of RPE cells with the preclinical vector results in dose-dependent expression of the *hRPE65* cDNA without any significant cell toxicity/death (Bennicelli et al. 2008).

2.3.5 Preclinical (In Vivo) Data

Two groups simultaneously explored the possibility of gene augmentation therapy-based rescue in the *RPE65* dog model using AAV. One team was at the University of Pennsylvania with collaborators in New York and Florida (Acland et al. 2001, 2005) and the other at the University of Missouri with collaborators at the University of Western Australia (Narfstrom et al. 2003a, b, c, 2005). Similar studies were also later carried out in Europe (Rolling et al. 2006) and, later, at the Children's Hospital of Philadelphia (CHOP) in collaboration with the University of Missouri (Bennicelli et al. 2008).

The results of all groups showed dramatic restoration of vision after a single subretinal delivery of AAV.RPE65. A summary of the results follows. All institutional and national guidelines for the care and use of laboratory animals were followed. All dogs evaluated, which received a successful subretinal injection before the age of 14 months, showed treatment success for rod and cone function by ERG (Bennicelli et al. 2008; Acland et al. 2001, 2005; Narfstrom et al. 2003a, b, c, 2005). Visual behavior could be observed by 1 month after vector administration. Improvement in visual function was dramatic and persisted for the duration of the study (Bennicelli et al. 2008; Acland et al. 2001, 2005; Narfstrom et al. 2003a, b, c, 2005). Behavioral studies showed a significantly improved ability of animals that received the appropriate subretinal dose to navigate through an obstacle course. Ocular motility studies showed signs that the treatment significantly reduced nystagmus corresponding to improved fixation and visual acuity (Jacobs et al. 2006, 2009).

Dogs were euthanized and enucleated at various times after treatment, ranging from 3 months to more than 11 years (Acland et al. 2005; Bennicelli et al. 2008; Cideciyan et al. 2013; Narfstrom et al. 2003c) to demonstrate persistence of transgene expression. Both transgene expression and efficacy persisted through the longest time points. These are significant periods of time with respect to both safety and stability of expression.

In studies of Rpe65−/− mice, AAV2 vectors did not initially result in efficacy after subretinal injection of AAV2.hRPE65. Efficacy was not identified unless AAV serotype 1 vectors were used (Dejneka et al. 2004b). With AAV1 vectors, subretinal injection performed up to 4 months of age resulted in significantly enhanced restoration of function whereas subretinal injection in aged mice (>15 months old) resulted in only minimal improvement in function (Jacobson et al. 2005). Subsets of eyes were analyzed both biochemically (for 11-cis retinal) and histologically for presence of RPE65 protein and the production of rhodopsin. Rhodopsin was identified only in the subretinally injected eyes (Dejneka et al. 2004b). This finding is important as this molecule would not be formed in these animals without delivery of the RPE65 protein and its subsequent role in production of the rhodopsin moiety, 11-cis retinal (Redmond et al. 1998). In the animals in which rhodopsin was produced, the ERG of the injected eye resembled that seen in normal sighted animals. In contrast, the control-injected eyes had little or no recordable responses even to the highest stimulus intensities.

It was not until the transgene cassette was further optimized (introduction of a Kozak sequence, etc.) that AAV2-mediated rescue was observed in Rpe65−/− mice (Bennicelli et al. 2008). It was fortunate that the initial studies in LCA2 were carried out in canine models rather than murine models, as investigators might not have proceeded to work with canine models after seeing negative results in the *Rpe65−/−* mice!

2.4 Description of the Trial

2.4.1 Results of the Studies at the Children's Hospital of Philadelphia (CHOP)

All procedures followed were in accordance with the ethical standards of the responsible committee on human experimentation (institutional and national) and with the Helsinki Declaration of 1975, as revised in 2000 (http://www.wma.net/en/30publications/10policies/b3/). Our study was the first to enroll pediatric subjects in a gene therapy trial for a nonlethal disease (see below). The informed consent/assent process was carried out through a series of discussions and review of written and auditory materials. Informed consent or assent and parental permission was obtained from all subjects included in the study.

Participants were injected subretinally in the eye with worse vision in a dose-escalation study. Doses ranged from 1.5×10^{10} to 1.5×10^{11} vector genomes (vg) of the AAV2 vector (AAV2.hRPE65v2) (16, 18). Each one of the subjects showed improvement in multiple measures of retinal and visual function in the injected eye. Most of the subjects showed improvement in full-field light sensitivity and pupillary light reflex (PLR) (Maguire et al. 2008, 2009). About half of the subjects showed significant improvement in visual acuity, and all showed a trend toward improvement in visual fields. Five of the 12 patients (including all pediatric subjects age 8–11 years) developed the ability to navigate a standardized obstacle course (Maguire et al. 2008, 2009). The improvements were measured as early as 2 weeks after treatment and persisted through the latest time point (now >6.5 years for the initial subjects) (Maguire et al. 2008, 2009; Simonelli et al. 2010). Functional magnetic resonance imaging (fMRI) studies carried out in subjects after they had received the injection also showed that the visual cortex became responsive to retinal input after this unilateral gene therapy, even after prolonged visual deprivation (Ashtari et al. 2011). Both the retina and the visual cortex became far more sensitive to dim light and lower-contrast stimuli.

The success of the unilateral injections begged the question of whether further benefit would result from injection of the second eye. The main concern had been that the initial injection would incite a harmful immune response and that this would prevent benefit in the second injected eye and/or result in inflammation in the initially injected eye. Prior to evaluating the safety of AAV2-hRPE65v2 in humans, sequential subretinal readministration of high-dose (1.5E11 vg) AAV2-hRPE65v2 was tested in both Briard (affected) dogs as well as unaffected nonhuman primates (NHPs) that had been previously systemically exposed to AAV (Amado et al. 2010). There were no safety concerns with respect to readministration in either the initially injected eye or the second (contralateral) eye (Amado et al. 2010). An additional preclinical toxicology study, designed in consultation with FDA, examined the effects of readministration in unaffected NHPs of doses that were twofold and fivefold higher than the high dose of the Phase 1 human trial and 20-fold and 50-fold higher than the low-dose cohort. There was no indication of ocular toxicity, and there were no test article-related clinical signs of systemic toxicity (Amado et al. 2010). Thus, the results from the animal studies were reassuring with respect to the potential safety of readministration to the contralateral eye in humans.

Because results from animal studies are not always predictive of the effects in humans, the human readministration studies proceeded cautiously. This "follow-on" study entailed injection of a single dose/volume (10^{13} vg in 300 μl) of AAV2.hRPE65v2 to the second (contralateral) eye. As an extra precaution and in order to optimize the risk-benefit ratio, each of the first three patients receiving readministration was an adult and was deemed least likely to benefit, based on the number of remaining retinal photoreceptors in each eye. There was a 2-month stagger between each of the 3 patients, and each patient was evaluated weekly in the clinic using a battery of ophthalmic and immunologic studies during the initial 3-month follow-up phase (Bennett et al. 2012).

Clinical examinations, immunology studies, and retinal/visual function tests following the initial contralateral eye injections demonstrated the safety and efficacy of the bilateral approach in the first three individuals, even with a delay between vector administrations (Bennett et al. 2012), consistent with findings in nonclinical studies (Amado et al. 2010). Administration of AAV2-hRPE65v2 to the contralateral eye was well tolerated; there were no cytotoxic T-cell responses to either vector (AAV2) or transgene product (RPE65) in any of the subjects. Neutralizing antibody (NAb) responses to AAV2 and RPE65 protein remained at or close to baseline in the postoperative period (Bennett et al. 2012). Most importantly, each one of the subjects showed improvements in retinal and visual function, including the finding that two of the subjects who had previously been unable to navigate the mobility course became able to complete the course accurately in dim light (Fig. 2.5) (Bennett et al. 2012). The follow-on study has proceeded to enroll the remaining subjects eligible for participation (Bennett et al., unpublished data).

2.4.2 The Approval Process

In the USA, there are a number of regulatory hurdles that must be negotiated before embarking on a gene therapy clinical trial. The first steps included a "Pre-Investigational New Device (IND) meeting" with the US Food Drug Administration (FDA) and a review by the NIH Office of Biologic Activities (OBA) Recombinant DNA Advisory Committee (RAC). The NIH established the RAC in 1974 in response to public concerns regarding the safety of manipulating DNA. This committee is a federal advisory committee that provides recommendations related to basic and clinical research involving recombinant or synthetic nucleic acid molecules. The NIH RAC decides whether to hold a public review. Because our trial was the first to enroll children (a "vulnerable population") for a gene therapy study for a nonlethal disease, it was the subject of focus of a public meeting (see Human gene transfer protocol #0510-740, http://www.webconferences.com/nihoba/13_dec_2005.html). Reviews from the hospital Institutional Biosafety Committee (IBC) and Institutional Review Board (IRB) followed along with review and approval

from a Data Safety Monitoring Board (DSMB), and finally, the Investigational New Device (IND) was submitted and reviewed by the US Food and Drug Administration (FDA). A similar process was carried out in order to undertake the follow-on study and the Phase III clinical trial that is in process.

2.4.3 The Manufacturing

AAV2-hRPE65v2 employs AAV as a delivery vehicle for normal human *RPE65*. The gene therapy material used at CHOP was manufactured under current Good Manufacturing Practices (cGMP) using a characterized HEK 293 cell line. The method that was used to generate the recombinant AAV vectors involved co-transfection of HEK 293 cells with three plasmids: the AAV vector plasmid pAAV.CMV.CβA.hRPE65v2 (containing the CBA-hRPE65 expression cassette flanked by AAV2 inverted terminal repeats (ITRs)) (Bennicelli et al. 2008), an AAV packaging plasmid providing AAV2 rep and cap sequences required for vector packaging, and an adenovirus helper plasmid providing minimal adenovirus sequences required for recombinant AAV packaging (E2A and E4 genes and RNA from serotype 2 adenovirus). The vector was purified through microfluidization, filtration, cation-exchange chromatography, density gradient ultracentrifugation and final diafiltration into phosphate-buffered saline containing 0.001 % Pluronic F68 (Bennicelli et al. 2008; Maguire et al. 2008, 2009). The Pluronic prevents subsequent losses of vector to product contact surfaces during storage and administration and thus assures accurate dosing (Bennicelli et al. 2008) (see above).

2.4.4 The First Subject

The first subject at CHOP was NP-01, a 26-year-old Caucasian mother of two children, and one of the three children in her family affected with LCA2. She and her siblings had been legally blind since birth. Subject NP-01 was referred by Dr. F. Simonelli, the Second University of Naples (SUN) in Italy. Molecular diagnosis of a mutation in the *RPE65* gene was initially performed at the Telethon Institute of Genetics and Medicine (TIGEM) and confirmed by the CLIA-approved Carver Laboratory at the University of Iowa (Maguire et al. 2008). The informed consent process occurred at both SUN and CHOP, and unilateral subretinal administration of AAV2-hRPE65v2 occurred at CHOP on October 11, 2007. Both SUN and CHOP carried out baseline and postinjection studies and found similar results. NP01 has been followed for 6.5 years since injection of her first eye.

NP-01 was also one of the first three subjects to participate in the CHOP follow-on (second eye readministration) study approximately 3.5 years after administration to her first eye (Table 2.1). She was 29 years of age at her second surgery (Bennett et al. 2012). NP01 was truly the pioneer for this study, volunteering as one of the first individuals for both initial administration and second eye administration studies. NP01 received the lowest dose in the Phase I escalation study (1.5E10 vg) and received the highest dose (1.5E11 vg) in the readministration study.

2.4.5   The Tests

Baseline and follow-up testing include a battery of safety assessments as well as child-friendly assessments of retinal and visual function. Testing included the following:

2.4.5.1 Safety Assessments

Ophthalmic exams included vision testing, slit lamp biomicroscopy, intraocular pressure measurements, fundoscopy with indirect ophthalmoscopic exam, fundus photography, and fundus biomicroscopy (optical coherence tomography (OCT)). Kinetic visual fields were measured using Goldmann perimetry and electroretinograms (ERGs) were performed. The presence and character of any nystagmus was monitored. Systemic safety was measured using complete blood counts and serum chemistries (including liver and renal function panels). Peripheral blood and tear fluid were evaluated for evidence of vector exposure through quantitative (Q)-PCR.

Immunologic studies evaluated humoral response to the transgene product (the RPE65 protein), neutralizing antibodies to V2, and T-cell responses to the V2 capsid and to the RPE65 protein (Maguire et al. 2008, 2009).

2.4.5.2 Retinal and Visual Function Assessments

Visual acuity was measured with Early Treatment Diabetic Retinopathy Study (ETDRS) testing. Goldmann perimetry was used to measure visual fields. Pupillary light reflex (PLR) responses were recorded simultaneously in both eyes with a Procyon P2000 pupillometer and PupilFit4 software (Monmouthshire, UK). Test paradigms involved both unilateral stimuli and stimuli that were presented alternatively to one eye and then the other. Light sensitivity was evaluated using full-field threshold sensitivity testing (FST) and stimuli included white, red, and blue lights. Characteristics of nystagmus were evaluated by videotaping the eye movements for qualitative clinical analysis of the subject's oscillation and strabismus. Navigational abilities were evaluated using a standardized "obstacle course." This mobility test is designed to mimic the types of obstacles that a visually impaired individual must navigate on a daily basis. The subject enters the course at a designated spot and follows arrows on the tiles such that there are a series of choices of movements to maneuver around or over the obstacles. Performance under different light levels was evaluated (Fig. 2.5). The size of the test course is within the constraints of the clinical examining room, and the course was modified from session to session so that the subject could not "learn" the course (Maguire et al. 2008, 2009).

2.4.5.3 CHOP Results: Phase I/II Trial Safety Profile

Immunologic responses were benign and no serious adverse events occurred relating to the vector. Serum antibodies to the *RPE65* transgene product were not detected after vector administration. There were mild increases in serum neutralizing antibodies to AAV2 immediately postinjection in some individuals; however, levels diminished quickly and returned to baseline levels by day 365 after vector administration. The vector was found in samples of tears and blood only transiently after surgery.

Except for the first subject, the target area was the macula for those individuals who had sufficient retinal cells in this region. There were three individuals with substantial atrophy in the macula and in whom macular exposure was thus limited. There were some (not unexpected) surgical complications, including a macular hole in one of the subjects at d14 (despite significant improvement in retinal/visual function). A foveal dehiscence was noted at the time of injection in another individual as some of the vector escaped from the foveal defect.

All of the retinal detachments had resolved by first postoperative visit (within 14 h after surgery), and foveal abnormalities were noted in only the one patient (NP02, see above), with optical coherence tomography. The foveal dehiscence in patient CH10 had completely resolved with no evidence of a macular hole after surgery at the first assessment. All the other postoperative retinal assessments were unremarkable. In order to minimize future surgical complications (such as macular hole), the surgical procedure was modified to minimize the stress on the fovea. The PIs of the other clinical trials were contacted immediately and advised about steps to minimize this potential complication.

Efficacy

All 12 individuals in the CHOP Phase I/II study reported improved vision in dimly lit environments in the injected eyes starting by 2 weeks after surgery. Improvements in visual acuity were substantial in more than half the subjects. The improvement was not associated with age; however, the baseline visual acuity was higher in children than in adults (Maguire et al. 2008, 2009).

Although visual field tests in patients with severe impairment show substantial variability, there was a trend to improvement and the enlargements exceeded the variation in the contralateral non-injected eye. The extent of improvement in visual fields correlated roughly with the amount of salvageable retina that was targeted (Maguire et al. 2008, 2009).

All individuals had bilaterally diminished full-field sensitivity at baseline. After injection, a large interocular difference (i.e., difference in sensitivity between injected and non-injected eyes) in full-field sensitivity was noted (Fig. 2.3). Only the injected eyes showed improved sensitivity. Improvements in full-field sensitivity were

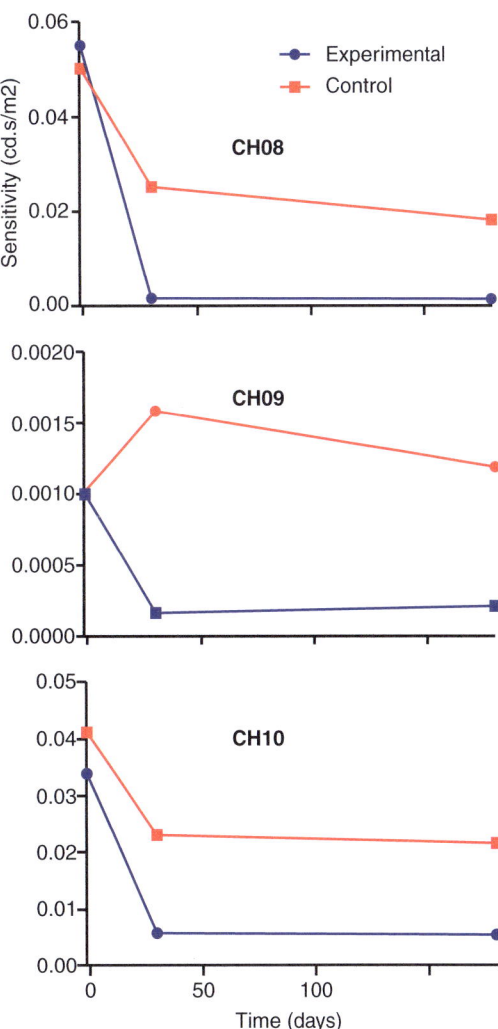

Fig. 2.3 Examples of before and after FSTs in the first three children enrolled in the Phase I study at the Children's Hospital of Philadelphia (Maguire et al. 2009). Note the increase in sensitivity of the experimental (injected) eye by day 30 after subretinal injection. Sensitivity is maintained through the latest time point shown (day 180). There can be changes in sensitivity of the uninjected (control) eye; however, these are not as large or as stable as those in the injected eye. Day 0, day of subretinal injection

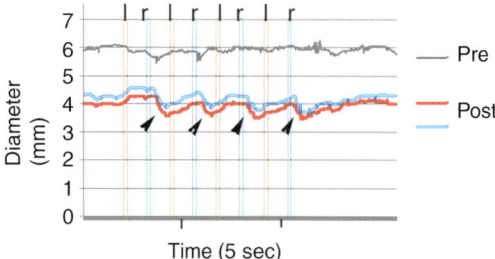

Fig. 2.4 Example of improvement in pupillary light reflex after subretinal injection of AAV2.hRPE65v2. Pupillary light reflex before (pre) intervention is shown in gray for the right pupil for one subject enrolled in the Phase 1 clinical trial at The Children's Hospital of Philadelphia (Maguire et al. 2008). Pupillary light reflex after intervention in the right eye (post) is shown in blue for the right pupil and red for the left pupil. *Arrowheads* indicate the improved responses only in the treated (right) eye. *Vertical dashed columns* indicate the stimuli presented to the left (l) vs right (r) eye

substantial in the youngest patients, who gained several log units of sensitivity (Maguire et al. 2009).

Pupillary responses improved in the injected eyes of all 11 individuals tested.

When the injected eye was illuminated with light, both pupils constricted; when the control, non-injected eye was illuminated with light, minimum constriction of the pupil was seen (Fig. 2.4). There were substantial differences between the injected and control eyes in the amplitude and velocity of constriction (Maguire et al. 2009).

The amplitude and frequency of nystagmus was reduced in several of the subjects after intervention of one eye. In some cases, this may have contributed to improved visual acuity in the non-injected eye (Maguire et al. 2008, 2009; Simonelli et al. 2010).

When patients were tested for their ability to navigate a standardized obstacle course before administration of AAV2-hRPE65v2, the majority had great difficulty, especially in dim light, as assessed by the number of errors and time taken. After injection, all of the children (CH08, CH09, CH10, and NP15) given AAV2-hRPE65v2 had substantial improvement in their ambulation when using only their injected eye. They were unable to navigate the course accurately using their non-injected eye (Maguire

et al. 2009). Similarly some of the adults who were unable to complete the mobility test with their initially injected eye were able to complete the course after the second eye was treated (with higher-dose vector; Fig. 2.5).

All individuals tested with functional magnetic resonance imaging (fMRI) showed restoration of cortical responses based on the known anatomic connections between the retina and the visual cortex and the area of retinal exposure to the gene therapy reagent (Ashtari et al. 2011). fMRI testing confirmed the increased sensitivity of these individuals to light and to objects of reduced contrast (Ashtari et al. 2011).

CHOP Results: Phase I/II Follow-On Trial

Results from the first three subjects enrolled in the follow-on study have been published (Bennett et al. 2012). In those three individuals, all of whom were adults, there was no inflammation resulting from readministration of vector and immune responses were benign. The originally injected eye maintained the function it had gained after the first injection, and the second eye gained function as judged by pupillometry and full-field light sensitivity (Bennett et al. 2012). Two of the individuals had previously received a lower dose in their initially injected eyes. The data provided a suggestion of a dose effect, with the high-dose-treated eye showing even better function than the initially treated (low dose or medium dose) eye (Bennett et al. 2012). Two of the individuals who had received lower doses in their initially injected eyes became able to navigate the mobility course after their second eye was injected. fMRI testing also showed the predicted improvement in visual cortex activation (Bennett et al. 2012).

2.5   Future Plans at CHOP

At present, we are conducting a Phase III (pivotal) trial at CHOP. The goal is that AAV2-hRPE65v2 be approved as a drug for treatment of LCA2. This multicenter (CHOP and University of Iowa) Phase III study involves bilateral administration

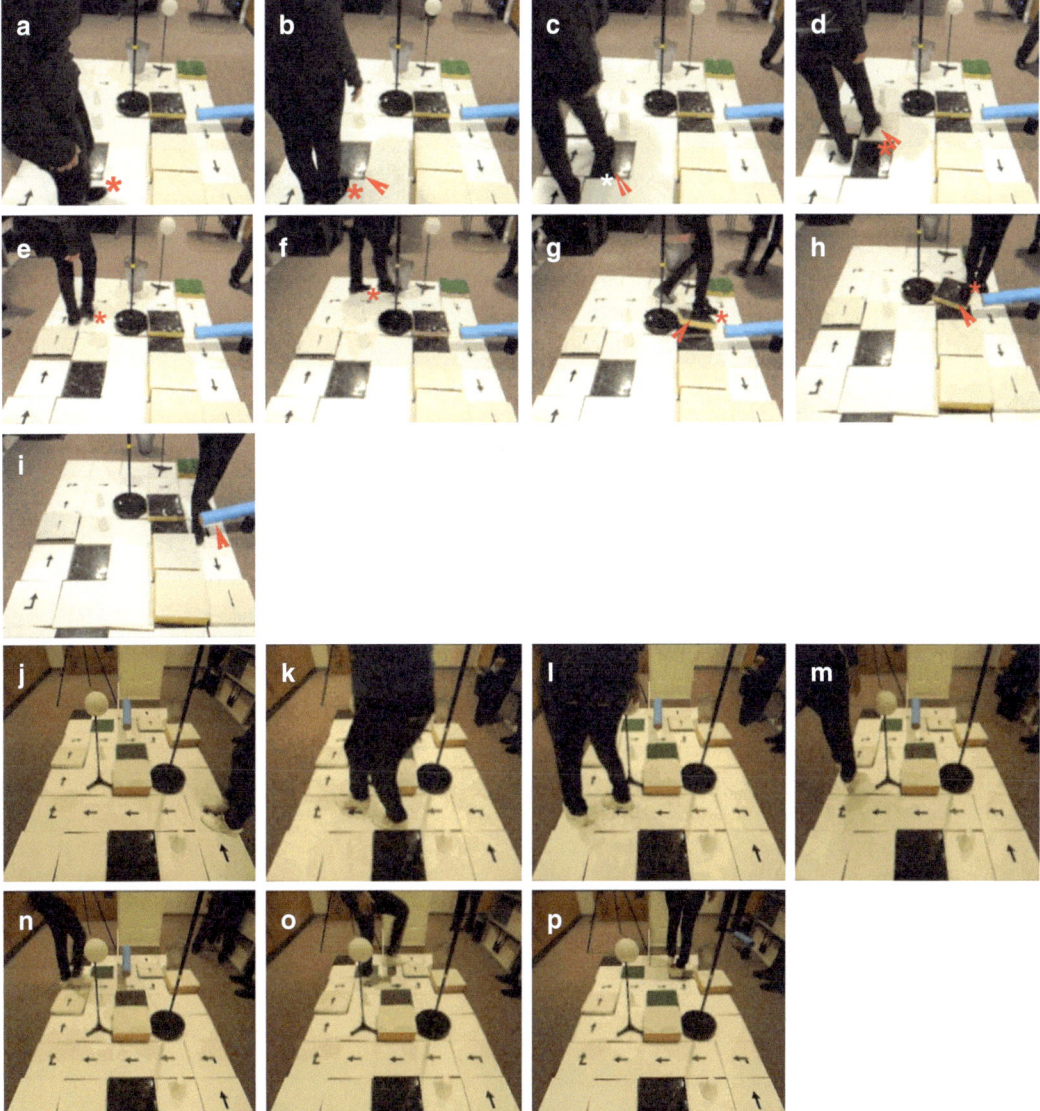

Fig. 2.5 Example of mobility test results, before and after readministration of AAV2.hRPE65v2. Frames from videos where subject NP01 undergoes obstacle course testing prior to (a–i) and 30 days following (j–p) intervention (Maguire et al. 2009). Light intensity was 50 lux for baseline testing and 5 lux for post-intervention testing. At baseline, NP01 goes off course repeatedly (*), collides with every obstacle (*arrowheads*), and takes 39 s to complete the course. After intervention, she completes the course in 14 s and does so without going off course or colliding with any obstacle

of AAV2.hRPE65v2 at 1.5E11 vg to the subretinal space in eligible individuals ages 3 years and higher. Subjects are randomized 2:1 to the intervention or control group, respectively. The individuals randomized to control crossover to the intervention group at year 1. Grading of primary endpoints is carried out by individuals masked as to whether the subjects have been assigned to the intervention vs the control arm of the study. Given maintenance of the current timeline, continued safety and efficacy, and no setbacks, such approval could be granted in 2016. All of the studies leading up to and including the Phase III trial stem from the efforts of a very large group of talented scientists who designed and carried out the relevant multifaceted studies. The success of translational studies depends not on the efforts of one person but instead on the integrated efforts of molecular geneticists, experts in animal models, astute clinicians, surgeons, geneticists, virologists, clinical coordinators, regulatory experts, administrators, data analysts, and, of course, the patients themselves.

Assuming that AAV2.hRPE65v2 is ultimately approved as a treatment for LCA2, we will undertake a training program for retinal surgeons on surgical details that could optimize the outcome. We hope that the CHOP data will pave the way for safe and rapid development of other gene-based interventions for inherited and acquired retinal disease. The "de-risking" of subretinal AAV2 delivery (at least for doses up to 1.5E11 vg of purified vector) may allow more rapid development of additional retinal gene therapy strategies. Of course, each new variable will have to be approached cautiously.

In presenting our data, we believe that we have set an example of the importance of highlighting not only the exciting efficacy data but have also highlighted complications. It is from the complications that we can all learn how to develop the optimal treatment approaches and to avoid untoward events in the future. We have shared and continue to share our experiences on a wide range of topics, including surgical approaches, vector selection data, and issues relating to vulnerable subjects with the goal of helping to expand the opportunities to rescue vision in individuals of all ages. We strive to present our data and the most logical explanations without political agenda. Most importantly, we believe that we have set an example of how individuals with complementary talents and experience in a large team can work safely, efficiently, and persistently together toward the goal of generating not only a safe treatment for a blinding disease but also to create a path whereby treatments can be developed for other blinding diseases.

Compliance with Ethical Requirements
Conflict of Interest Jean Bennett and her husband and collaborator, Albert M. Maguire, are coinventors of a patent for a method to treat or slow the development of blindness (US Patent 8,147,823 B2; April 3, 2012), but both waived financial interest in this technology in 2002. JB serves on a data safety monitoring board for Sanofi and as a scientific advisor to Spark Therapeutics and Avalanche Biotechnologies, Inc. She is a cofounder of GenSight Biologics.

No animal or human studies were carried out by the author for this chapter.

References

Acland GM, Aguirre GD, Ray J, Zhang Q, Aleman TS, Cideciyan AV, Pearce-Kelling SE, Anand V, Zeng Y, Maguire AM, Jacobson SG, Hauswirth WW, Bennett J (2001) Gene therapy restores vision in a canine model of childhood blindness. Nat Genet 28(1):92–95

Acland GM, Aguirre GD, Bennett J, Aleman TS, Cideciyan AV, Bennicelli J, Dejneka NS, Pearce-Kelling SE, Maguire AM, Palczewski K, Hauswirth WW, Jacobson SG (2005) Long-term restoration of rod and cone vision by single dose rAAV-mediated gene transfer to the retina in a canine model of childhood blindness. Mol Ther 12(6):1072–1082. doi:10.1016/j.ymthe.2005.08.008, S1525-0016(05)01561-3 [pii]

Aguirre G, Baldwin V, Pearce-Kelling S, Narfstrom K, Ray K, Acland G (1998) Congenital stationary night blindness in the dog: common mutation in the RPE65 gene indicates founder effect. Mol Vis 4:23

Aleman TS, Jacobson SG, Chico JD, Scott ML, Cheung AY, Windsor EA, Furushima M, Redmond TM, Bennett J, Palczewski K, Cideciyan AV (2004) Impairment of the transient pupillary light reflex in Rpe65(−/−) mice and humans with leber congenital amaurosis. Invest Ophthalmol Vis Sci 45(4):1259–1271

Ali RR, Reichel MB, Thrasher AJ, Levinsky RJ, Kinnon C, Kanuga N, Hunt DM, Bhattacharya SS (1996) Gene transfer into the mouse retina mediated by an adeno-associated viral vector. Hum Mol Genet 5(5):591–594

Amado D, Mingozzi F, Hui D, Bennicelli J, Wei Z, Chen Y, Bote E, Grant R, Golden J, Narfstrom K, Syed N, Orlin S, Maguire A, High K, Bennett J (2010) Safety and efficacy of subretinal re-administration of an AAV2 vector in large animal models: implications for studies in humans. Sci Transl Med 2:21ra16

Ashtari M, Cyckowski LL, Monroe JF, Marshall KA, Chung DC, Auricchio A, Simonelli F, Leroy BP, Maguire AM, Shindler KS, Bennett J (2011) The human visual cortex responds to gene therapy-mediated recovery of retinal function. J Clin Invest 121(6):2160–2168. doi:10.1172/JCI57377, 57377 [pii]

Bainbridge JW, Smith AJ, Barker SS, Robbie S, Henderson R, Balaggan K, Viswanathan A, Holder GE, Stockman A, Tyler N, Petersen-Jones S, Bhattacharya SS, Thrasher AJ, Fitzke FW, Carter BJ, Rubin GS, Moore AT, Ali RR (2008) Effect of gene therapy on visual function in Leber's congenital amaurosis. N Engl J Med 358(21):2231–2239

Banin E, Bandah-Rozenfeld D, Obolensky A, Cideciyan AV, Aleman TS, Marks-Ohana D, Sela M, Boye S, Sumaroka A, Roman AJ, Schwartz SB, Hauswirth WW, Jacobson SG, Hemo I, Sharon D (2010) Molecular anthropology meets genetic medicine to treat blindness in the North African Jewish population: human gene therapy initiated in Israel. Hum Gene Ther 21(12):1749–1757. doi:10.1089/hum.2010.047

Bennett J, Wilson J, Sun D, Forbes B, Maguire A (1994) Adenovirus vector-mediated in vivo gene transfer into adult murine retina. Invest Ophthalmol Vis Sci 35(5):2535–2542

Bennett J, Tanabe T, Sun D, Zeng Y, Kjeldbye H, Gouras P, Maguire A (1996) Photoreceptor cell rescue in retinal degeneration (*rd*) mice by in vivo gene therapy. Nat Med 2(6):649–654

Bennett J, Duan D, Engelhardt JF, Maguire AM (1997) Real-time, noninvasive in vivo assessment of adeno-associated virus-mediated retinal transduction. Invest Ophthalmol Vis Sci 38(13):2857–2863

Bennett J, Ashtari M, Wellman J, Marshall KA, Cyckowski LL, Chung DC, McCague S, Pierce EA, Chen Y, Bennicelli JL, Zhu X, Ying GS, Sun J, Wright JF, Auricchio A, Simonelli F, Shindler KS, Mingozzi F, High KA, Maguire AM (2012) AAV2 gene therapy readministration in three adults with congenital blindness. Sci Transl Med 4(120):120ra115. doi:10.1126/scitranslmed.3002865, 4/120/120ra15 [pii]

Bennicelli J, Wright JF, Komaromy A, Jacobs JB, Hauck B, Zelenaia O, Mingozzi F, Hui D, Chung D, Rex TS, Wei Z, Qu G, Zhou S, Zeiss C, Arruda VR, Acland GM, Dell'Osso LF, High KA, Maguire AM, Bennett J (2008) Reversal of blindness in animal models of leber congenital amaurosis using optimized AAV2-mediated gene transfer. Mol Ther 16(3):458–465

Borras T, Tamm ER, Zigler JS Jr (1996) Ocular adenovirus gene transfer varies in efficiency and inflammatory response. Invest Ophthalmol Vis Sci 37(7):1282–1293

Carter BJ (1996) The promise of adeno-associated virus vectors. Nat Biotechnol 14:1725–1726

Cideciyan AV, Aleman TS, Boye SL, Schwartz SB, Kaushal S, Roman AJ, Pang JJ, Sumaroka A, Windsor EA, Wilson JM, Flotte TR, Fishman GA, Heon E, Stone EM, Byrne BJ, Jacobson SG, Hauswirth WW (2008) Human gene therapy for RPE65 isomerase deficiency activates the retinoid cycle of vision but with slow rod kinetics. Proc Natl Acad Sci U S A 105(39):15112–15117

Cideciyan AV, Hauswirth W, Aleman TS, Kaushal S, Schwartz SB, Boye SL, Windsor E, Conlon T, Sumaroka A, Pang JJ, Roman AJ, Byrne B, Jacobson SG (2009a) Human RPE65 gene therapy for leber congenital amaurosis: persistence of early visual improvements and safety at one year. Hum Gene Ther 20(9):999–1004

Cideciyan AV, Hauswirth WW, Aleman TS, Kaushal S, Schwartz SB, Boye SL, Windsor EA, Conlon TJ, Sumaroka A, Roman AJ, Byrne BJ, Jacobson SG (2009b) Vision 1 year after gene therapy for Leber's congenital amaurosis. N Engl J Med 361(7):725–727

Cideciyan AV, Jacobson SG, Beltran WA, Sumaroka A, Swider M, Iwabe S, Roman AJ, Olivares MB, Schwartz SB, Komaromy AM, Hauswirth WW, Aguirre GD (2013) Human retinal gene therapy for Leber congenital amaurosis shows advancing retinal degeneration despite enduring visual improvement. Proc Natl Acad Sci U S A. doi:10.1073/pnas.1218933110, 1218933110 [pii]

Cremers F, Brunsmann F, Berger W, van Kerkhoff E, van de Pol T, Wieringa B, Pawlowitzki I, Ropers H-H (1990) Cloning of the breakpoints of a deletion associated with choroideremia. Hum Genet 86:61–64

Dejneka N, Surace E, Aleman T, Cideciyan A, Lyubarsky A, Savchenko A, Redmond T, Tang W, Wei Z, Rex T, Glover E, Maguire A, Pugh E, Jacobson S, Bennett J (2004a) Fetal virus-mediated delivery of the human RPE65 gene rescues vision in a murine model of congenital retinal blindness. Mol Ther 9:182–188

Dejneka NS, Surace EM, Aleman TS, Cideciyan AV, Lyubarsky A, Savchenko A, Redmond TM, Tang W, Wei Z, Rex TS, Glover E, Maguire AM, Pugh EN Jr, Jacobson SG, Bennett J (2004b) In utero gene therapy rescues vision in a murine model of congenital blindness. Mol Ther 9(2):182–188

Dryja TP, McGee T, Reichel E, Hahn L, Cowley B, Yandell DW, Sandberg M, Berson EL (1990) A point mutation of the rhodopsin gene in one form of retinitis pigmentosa. Nature 343:364–366

Flannery JG, Zolotukhin S, Vaquero MI, LaVail MM, Muzyczka N, Hauswirth WW (1997) Efficient photoreceptor-targeted gene expression in vivo by recombinant adeno-associated virus. Proc Natl Acad Sci U S A 94(13):6916–6921

Gu SM, Thompson DA, Srikumari CR, Lorenz B, Finckh U, Nicoletti A, Murthy KR, Rathmann M, Kumaramanickavel G, Denton MJ, Gal A (1997) Mutations in RPE65 cause autosomal recessive childhood-onset severe retinal dystrophy. Nat Genet 17(2):194–197

Hauswirth WW, Aleman TS, Kaushal S, Cideciyan AV, Schwartz SB, Wang L, Conlon TJ, Boye SL, Flotte TR, Byrne BJ, Jacobson SG (2008) Treatment of leber congenital amaurosis due to RPE65 mutations by ocular subretinal injection of adeno-associated virus gene vector: short-term results of a phase I trial. Hum Gene Ther 19(10):979–990. doi:10.1089/hum.2008.107

Hoffman LM, Maguire AM, Bennett J (1997) Cell-mediated immune response and stability of intraocular transgene expression after adenovirus-mediated delivery. Invest Ophthalmol Vis Sci 38(11):2224–2233

Humphries P, Farrar GJ, Kenna P, McWilliam P (1990) Retinitis pigmentosa: genetic mapping in X-linked and autosomal forms of the disease. Clin Genet 38(1):1–13

Jacobs J, Dell'Osso L, Hertle R, Acland G, Bennett J (2006) Eye movement recordings as an effectiveness indicator of gene therapy in RPE65-deficient canines: implications for the ocular motor system. Invest Ophthalmol Vis Sci 47(7):2865–2875

Jacobs JB, Dell'Osso LF, Wang ZI, Acland GM, Bennett J (2009) Using the NAFX to measure the effectiveness over time of gene therapy in canine LCA. Invest Ophthalmol Vis Sci 50(10):4685–4692

Jacobson SG, Aleman TS, Cideciyan AV, Sumaroka A, Schwartz SB, Windsor EA, Traboulsi EI, Heon E, Pittler SJ, Milam AH, Maguire AM, Palczewski K, Stone EM, Bennett J (2005) Identifying photoreceptors in blind eyes caused by RPE65 mutations: prerequisite for human gene therapy success. Proc Natl Acad Sci U S A 102(17):6177–6182

Jacobson S, Acland G, Aguirre GD, Aleman T, Schwartz S, Cideciyan A, Zeiss C, Komaromy A, Kaushal S, Roman A, Windsor E, Sumaroka A, Pearce-Kelling S, Conlon T, Boye S, Flotte T, Maguire A, Bennett J, Hauswirth W (2006) Safety of recombinant adeno-associated virus 2-RPE65 vector delivered by ocular subretinal injection. Mol Ther 13(6):1074–1084

Jacobson SG, Cideciyan AV, Ratnakaram R, Heon E, Schwartz SB, Roman AJ, Peden MC, Aleman TS, Boye SL, Sumaroka A, Conlon TJ, Calcedo R, Pang JJ, Erger KE, Olivares MB, Mullins CL, Swider M, Kaushal S, Feuer WJ, Iannaccone A, Fishman GA, Stone EM, Byrne BJ, Hauswirth WW (2012) Gene therapy for leber congenital amaurosis caused by RPE65 mutations: safety and efficacy in 15 children and adults followed up to 3 years. Arch Ophthalmol 130(1):9–24. doi:10.1001/archophthalmol.2011.298, archophthalmol.2011.298 [pii]

Jomary C, Vincent K, Grist J, Neal M, Jones S (1997) Rescue of photoreceptor function by AAV-mediated gene transfer in a mouse model of inherited retinal degeneration. Gene Ther 4:683–690

Li T, Adamian M, Roof DJ, Berson EL, Dryja TP, Roessler BJ, Davidson BL (1994) In vivo transfer of a reporter gene to the retina mediated by an adenoviral vector. Investig Ophthalmol Vis Sci 35(5):2543–2549

Lorenz B, Gyurus P, Preising M, Bremser D, Gu S, Andrassi M, Gerth C, Gal A (2000) Early-onset severe rod-cone dystrophy in young children with RPE65 mutations. Invest Ophthalmol Vis Sci 41(9):2735–2742

Maguire AM, Bennett J, Nickle A, Aguirre G, Acland G (1995) Adenovirus-mediated gene transfer to canine retinal photoreceptors: effects of inflammation. Invest Ophthalmol Vis Sci 36(4):S777

Maguire AM, Simonelli F, Pierce EA, Pugh EN Jr, Mingozzi F, Bennicelli J, Banfi S, Marshall KA, Testa F, Surace EM, Rossi S, Lyubarsky A, Arruda VR, Konkle B, Stone E, Sun J, Jacobs J, Dell'Osso L, Hertle R, Ma JX, Redmond TM, Zhu X, Hauck B, Zelenaia O, Shindler KS, Maguire MG, Wright JF, Volpe NJ, McDonnell JW, Auricchio A, High KA, Bennett J (2008) Safety and efficacy of gene transfer for Leber's congenital amaurosis. N Engl J Med 358(21):2240–2248

Maguire AM, High KA, Auricchio A, Wright JF, Pierce EA, Testa F, Mingozzi F, Bennicelli JL, Ying GS, Rossi S, Fulton A, Marshall KA, Banfi S, Chung DC, Morgan JI, Hauck B, Zelenaia O, Zhu X, Raffini L, Coppieters F, De Baere E, Shindler KS, Volpe NJ, Surace EM, Acerra C, Lyubarsky A, Redmond TM, Stone E, Sun J, McDonnell JW, Leroy BP, Simonelli F, Bennett J (2009)

Age-dependent effects of RPE65 gene therapy for Leber's congenital amaurosis: a phase 1 dose-escalation trial. Lancet 374(9701):1597–1605

Marlhens F, Bareil C, Friffoin J-M, Zrenner E, Amalric P, Eliaou C, Liu S-Y, Harris E, Redmond TM, Arnaud B, Claustres M, Hamel CP (1997) Mutations in RPE65 cause Leber's congenital amaurosis. Nat Genet 17:139–141

Morimura H, Fishman GA, Grover S, Fulton A, Berson E, Dryja T (1998) Mutations in the RPE65 gene in patients with autosomal recessive retinitis pigmentosa or Leber congenital amaurosis. Proc Natl Acad Sci U S A 95:3088–3093

Narfstrom K, Wrigstad A, Nilsson S (1989) The Briard dogs: a new animal model of congenital stationary night blindness. Br J Ophthalmol 73:750–756

Narfstrom K, Ehinger B, Bruun A (2001) Immuno-histochemical studies of cone photoreceptors and cells of the inner retina in feline rod-cone degeneration. Vet Ophthalmol 4:141–145

Narfstrom K, Bragadottir R, Redmond TM, Rakoczy PE, van Veen T, Bruun A (2003a) Functional and structural evaluation after AAV.RPE65 gene transfer in the canine model of Leber's congenital amaurosis. Adv Exp Med Biol 533:423–430

Narfstrom K, Katz ML, Bragadottir R, Seeliger M, Boulanger A, Redmond TM, Caro L, Lai CM, Rakoczy PE (2003b) Functional and structural recovery of the retina after gene therapy in the RPE65 null mutation dog. Invest Ophthalmol Vis Sci 44(4):1663–1672

Narfstrom K, Katz ML, Ford M, Redmond TM, Rakoczy E, Bragadottir R (2003c) In vivo gene therapy in young and adult RPE65−/− dogs produces long-term visual improvement. J Hered 94(1):31–37

Narfstrom K, Vaegan KM, Bragadottir R, Rakoczy EP, Seeliger M (2005) Assessment of structure and function over a 3-year period after gene transfer in RPE65−/− dogs. Doc Ophthalmol 111(1):39–48. doi:10.1007/s10633-005-3159-0

Nathans J, Hogness DS (1984) Isolation and nucleotide sequence of the gene encoding human rhodopsin. Proc Natl Acad Sci U S A 81:4851–4855

Pang JJ, Chang B, Hawes NL, Hurd RE, Davisson MT, Li J, Noorwez SM, Malhotra R, McDowell JH, Kaushal S, Hauswirth WW, Nusinowitz S, Thompson DA, Heckenlively JR (2005) Retinal degeneration 12 (rd12): a new, spontaneously arising mouse model for human Leber congenital amaurosis (LCA). Mol Vis 11:152–162

Perrault I, Rozet J, Gerber S, Ghazi I, Leowski C, Ducrow D, Souied E, Dufier J, Munnich A, Kaplan J (1999) Leber congenital amaurosis. Mol Genet Metab 68:200–208

Redmond T, Hamel C (2000) Genetic analysis of RPE65: from human disease to mouse model. Methods Enzymol 317:705–724

Redmond TM, Yu S, Lee E, Bok D, Hamasaki D, Chen N, Goletz P, Ma JX, Crouch RK, Pfeifer K (1998) Rpe65 is necessary for production of 11-cis-vitamin A in the retinal visual cycle. Nat Genet 20(4):344–351

RetNet (2014) http://www.sph.uth.tmc.edu/RetNet

Rojas-Burke J (2011) Oregon girl gets gene therapy to prevent blindness. The Oregonian, 16 Feb 2011

Rolling F, Le Meur G, Stieger K, Smith AJ, Weber M, Deschamps JY, Nivard D, Mendes-Madeira A, Provost N, Pereon Y, Cherel Y, Ali RR, Hamel C, Moullier P, Rolling F (2006) Gene therapeutic prospects in early onset of severe retinal dystrophy: restoration of vision in RPE65 Briard dogs using an AAV serotype 4 vector that specifically targets the retinal pigmented epithelium. Bull Mem Acad R Med Belg 161(10–12):497–508; discussion 508–499

Simonelli F, Ziviello C, Testa F, Rossi S, Fazzi E, Bianchi PE, Fossarello M, Signorini S, Bertone C, Galantuomo S, Brancati F, Valente EM, Ciccodicola A, Rinaldi E, Auricchio A, Banfi S (2007) Clinical and molecular genetics of Leber's congenital amaurosis: a multicenter study of Italian patients. Invest Ophthalmol Vis Sci 48(9):4284–4290

Simonelli F, Maguire AM, Testa F, Pierce EA, Mingozzi F, Bennicelli JL, Rossi S, Marshall K, Banfi S, Surace EM, Sun J, Redmond TM, Zhu X, Shindler KS, Ying GS, Ziviello C, Acerra C, Wright JF, McDonnell JW, High KA, Bennett J, Auricchio A (2010) Gene therapy for Leber's congenital amaurosis is safe and effective through 1.5 years after vector administration. Mol Ther 18(3):643–650

Thompson DA, Janecke AR, Lange J, Feathers KL, Hubner CA, McHenry CL, Stockton DW, Rammesmayer G, Lupski JR, Antinolo G, Ayuso C, Baiget M, Gouras P, Heckenlively JR, den Hollander A, Jacobson SG, Lewis RA, Sieving PA, Wissinger B, Yzer S, Zrenner E, Utermann G, Gal A (2005) Retinal degeneration associated with RDH12 mutations results from decreased 11-cis retinal synthesis due to disruption of the visual cycle. Hum Mol Genet 14(24):3865–3875. doi:10.1093/hmg/ddi411, ddi411 [pii]

Vandenberghe L, Bell P, Maguire A, Xiao R, Hopkins T, McMenamin D, Munden R, Grant R, Bennett J, Wilson J (2013) AAV9 targets cone photoreceptors in non-human primates. PLoS One 8(1):e53463. doi:10.1371/journal.pone.0053463

Veske A, Nilsson S, Narfstrom K, Gal A (1999) Retinal dystrophy of Swedish briard/briard-beagle dogs is due to a 4-bp deletion in RPE65. Genomics 57(1):57–61

Wade N (1999) Patient dies while undergoing gene therapy. New York Times, 29 Sept 1999

Gene Therapy for Choroideremia

Alun R. Barnard, Markus Groppe,
and Robert E. MacLaren

3.1 Description of the Disease

Choroideremia (CHM; OMIM Phenotype MIM number: 303100; ICD10 code H31.2) may first have been described in the nineteenth century by the Austrian ophthalmologist Ludwig Mauthner (1872) who observed a striking pale colour of the fundus in an individual with very poor vision. This would occur as the result of exposure of the underlying white sclera, which is a characteristic and normally easily recognisable feature in the later stages of choroideremia (Fig. 3.1). At the time, he attributed this to a congenital absence of the majority of the choroid, probably caused by a developmental disorder (Mauthner 1872).

A.R. Barnard, PhD (✉)
Nuffield Laboratory of Ophthalmology,
Department of Clinical Neurosciences and Oxford
Biomedical Research Centre, University of Oxford,
The John Radcliffe Hospital, Oxford OX3 9DU, UK
e-mail: alun.barnard@eye.ox.ac.uk

M. Groppe, PhD, FRCOphth, FEBO
R.E. MacLaren, MB, ChB, DPhil, FRCOphth, FRCS
Nuffield Laboratory of Ophthalmology,
Department of Clinical Neurosciences and Oxford
Biomedical Research Centre, University of Oxford,
The John Radcliffe Hospital, Oxford OX3 9DU, UK

Moorfields Eye Hospital and NIHR Biomedical
Research Centre for Ophthalmology, London
EC1V 2PD, UK
e-mail: enquiries@eye.ox.ac.uk

Seemingly as a result of the barren appearance of the fundus, Mauthner named the condition 'chorioideremie', which is thought to be a combination of the ancient Greek 'erēmia', meaning barren land or desert, as a suffix to the stem word 'chorioid', a common alternative spelling of 'choroid' (also originally from ancient Greek words for skin, 'chorion', and form/type, 'eidos') (Myers 2006). Thus, the disease name means 'an area barren of choroid'. We now know that the name choroideremia, although an apt description of the clinical appearance of atrophy of the choroid at later stages of the disease, does not reflect the aetiology of the disease very well. This is an important consideration when developing therapeutic strategies (see below).

It is now understood that choroideremia is an X-linked recessive degenerative disease of the retina. The condition is gradually progressive in males; it begins with reduced night vision in adolescence and develops with a gradual loss of peripheral vision and blindness in middle age (MacDonald et al. 2009). Choroideremia is not thought to affect eye formation and early visual development, unlike Leber congenital amaurosis (LCA) and many other visual cycle disorders.

However, the RPE, retina and choroid do begin slowly to undergo atrophy at an early age. Although male patients generally maintain good visual acuity until the degeneration encroaches on the fovea, underlying changes in the retina can be identified in childhood and are associated with

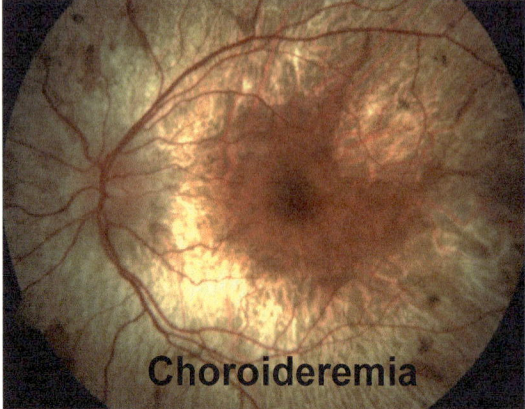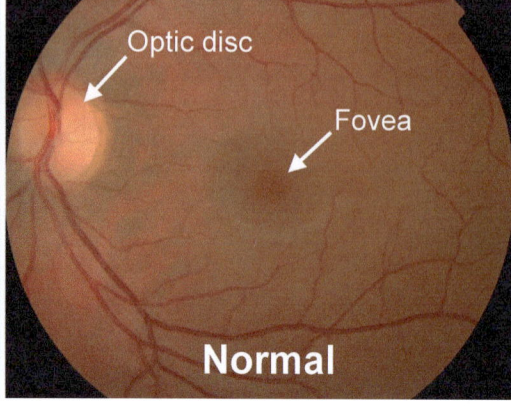

Fig. 3.1 A fundus photograph of a patient with advanced choroideremia (*left*) compared to a normal eye (*right*). The choroideremia eye has a characteristic pale appear-ance and there is a residual island of healthy tissue in the central macula and fovea

significant reductions in parafoveal retinal sensitivity as measured by psychophysical testing (Jacobson et al. 2006b). Disease progression is relatively slow and occurs after the period of visual development, and patients have largely unaffected vision particularly in early life. Because of this, the majority of patients would likely benefit from successful therapeutic intervention to preserve remaining vision, even at late stages of the disease.

Most female carriers exhibit characteristic pigmentary changes of the fundus when examined. The extent and impact of these changes likely depend on individual differences in the random process of X-inactivation. This commonly results in an even and fine distribution of affected and unaffected retinal pigment epithelium (RPE) cells across the eye. Individuals with this pattern remain predominantly asymptomatic in early years, but may develop reduced night vision in later years. In contrast, this process can also result in large areas of retina affected by choroideremia, and these rare but severe cases can lead to blindness in female carriers (Bonilha et al. 2008).

Choroideremia is classified as a rare disease; it has a predicted prevalence of approximately 1:50,000 in people of European descent, with the highest prevalence in northern Finland (Sankila et al. 1992). However, there are thought to be more than 500 affected male patients in the UK and around 3,000 throughout Europe (MacDonald et al. 2009), and thus, a significant patient population exists for this blinding disease which is currently lacking any major treatment options.

3.2 The Road to Treat Choroideremia

The team at Oxford is a mix of clinician-scientists and basic science researchers. This provides a good combination of skills, experience and opinions for generating important preclinical, translational studies and designing and implementing clinical trials. We became interested in developing a gene therapy trial for choroideremia because the disease is highly suitable for treatment using gene replacement therapy and because of the absence of any established treatments to stop or even slow the progression of retinal degeneration in the disease. The study chair (Robert MacLaren) assembled a trial study group which represents a collaboration between several leading academic centres, with various members contributing valuable individual expertise and experience.

The clinical research was further augmented by Miguel Seabra and his team, based at Imperial College London, who had conducted important work on elucidating the pathogenesis of choroideremia for a number of years, prior to the instigation of a gene therapy clinical trial. Importantly the trial also incorporates several ophthalmology centres across the UK including Moorfields Eye Hospital in London, which has probably the largest number of choroideremia patients in the world. Overall the trial brings together a mix of clinical and scientific expertise that is now being directed towards a Phase II clinical trial to assess gene therapy using AAV for choroideremia.

3.3 Major Milestones in the Discovery

3.3.1 Identification of the Gene

In the late twentieth century, it was discovered that choroideremia is caused by disruption of the *CHM* gene (OMIM Gene/Locus MIM number: 300390), which is located on the long arm of the X chromosome (Cremers et al. 1990; Merry et al. 1992). Although this was over a hundred years after the condition was first described, this discovery represented one of the very first disease-causing genes to be identified by positional cloning (identification based on precise chromosomal localisation) and enabled subsequent studies to be conducted that would provide new insights into the molecular mechanisms responsible for this disorder. In the following few years, it was determined that the *CHM* gene encodes Rab escort protein 1 (REP1), which is sometimes also referred to as component A of Rab geranylgeranyltransferase, and that the protein is expressed ubiquitously and found in all cell types and tissues throughout the body (Seabra et al. 1992a, b, 1993). Further work has shown that REP1 plays a role in fundamental cellular processes of intracellular vesicle trafficking and recycling, through its action on Rab GTPases (e.g. Seabra et al. 1992a, 1993, 1995; Pylypenko et al. 2003; Larijani et al. 2003; Tolmachova et al. 2006, 2010). Interestingly, most mammals (including man) produce a very similar protein to REP1, named REP2 (amino acid sequence 75 % identical, 90 % similar to

REP1, Cremers et al. 1994). REP2 is coded for by the gene CHML (choroideremia-like) which resides on chromosome 1 and is thought to have arisen from a retrogene insertion of the REP1 mRNA transcript sometime during vertebrate evolution (as evidenced by the lack of introns). REP2, like REP1, is expressed ubiquitously. Thus, loss of REP1 function can in theory be compensated for by the action of REP2. Why the action of REP2 appears to be able to compensate for the loss of function of REP1 in all cells and tissues, except the eye, remains an open question. However, it has been suggested that certain Rabs, such as Rab27a, are particularly important in the eye and are preferentially prenylated by REP1 (Tolmachova et al. 1999; Larijani et al. 2003) which might explain why REP2 is unable to compensate in the eyes of CHM patients over the long term.

3.3.2 Identification of the Delivery Vector

At the time of planning the choroideremia study, most ocular gene therapy clinical trials had used viral vectors based on the adeno-associated virus (AAV). This vector appeared to be a rational choice, but to assess whether an AAV-based vector was applicable for use in choroideremia, a number of issues had to be considered. The first issue was the amount of genetic material that can be placed into each viral particle. This limit (known as the packaging capacity) is thought to be <5 kilobases (kb) of single-stranded DNA for AAV vectors (Wu et al. 2010). Although this capacity is considered to be small, and a potential limitation of using AAV, it is more than sufficient to include the full coding sequence of REP1 (at 1.9 kb) while still allowing space for a choice of promoters and other regulatory elements.

Another important consideration is which cell types need to be targeted for gene replacement therapy (and which can or should be avoided). Related to this, an important question in choroideremia pathogenesis has been whether one cell type/tissue layer acts as a primary site of degeneration (which then leads to the demise of the other cell types/tissue layers) or if the disease appears in multiple cell types/tissue layers independently and/or simultaneously. The question is complicated by the fact that the three affected eye layers (choroid, photoreceptors and RPE) are highly interdependent. For example, genetically normal photoreceptors will degenerate secondary to loss of the pigment epithelium by any cause (for instance, in myopic and dry age-related macular degeneration), and the morphology and distribution of RPE cells will change in response to photoreceptor loss (e.g. in many forms of retinitis pigmentosa).

Recent work in a mouse model bearing a conditional knock out allele (*Chm^Flox*) that allows for the selective ablation of the *Chm* gene in a particular cell/tissue type is very relevant to this question. Without going into specific details, these studies found that there is an inherent, independent and cell-autonomous need for REP1 function in both the neurosensory retina and RPE cells, meaning that both the layers could be considered primary sites of the disease (Tolmachova et al. 2006, 2010). Importantly, these molecular-genetic animal studies are supported by observations of choroideremia pathology based on human data. In human female carriers, skewed X-inactivation across the retinal layers can leave affected clones of photoreceptors against normal pigment epithelial cells, and histological post-mortem specimens suggest that photoreceptors degenerate independently of the retinal pigment epithelium (Flannery et al. 1990; Syed et al. 2001; Bonilha et al. 2008). There is also evidence from optical coherence tomography (OCT) scans of male choroideremia patients that the photoreceptor layer thins in advance of degeneration of the pigment epithelium (Jacobson et al. 2006b).

Overall, the data suggest using a REP1 expressing vector that targets both the photoreceptor layer and the retinal pigment epithelium, but further refinement might also be necessary. Since the early stages of choroideremia are manifest by loss of night vision and central cone-mediated vision is preserved until very late stages of the disease, it seems reasonable to assume that rods are affected significantly more than cones. For reasons that are not completely clear, cones are known to be dependent on surrounding rods and any genetic condition that causes rod death will also lead to complete loss of cones in a centripetal pattern as a secondary phenomenon. In a post-mortem analysis of the retina from an X-linked carrier female, apparently normal REP1 deficient cones could be identified within regions containing REP1 expressing rods (Syed et al. 2001). The differential expression of REP1 in these two photoreceptor subclasses results from differential X-inactivation (Reese et al. 1995) and provides further evidence that cones may exist without REP1 when surrounded by rods. It therefore seems reasonable to assume that cone death may be occurring as a phenomenon secondary to loss of rods and retinal pigment epithelium, rather than a dependency on REP1. Hence, from a safety perspective, it might actually be better to avoid transduction of cone cells as much as possible.

The relative importance of REP1 deficiency in the choroidal layers has been not dealt with comprehensively in the animal models. Human studies have been more informative, and observations from post-mortem carrier females show no focal loss or abnormalities of the choroid except underlying areas of severe retinal degeneration (Syed et al. 2001) which suggests that the choroidal vascular system is not dependent on REP1. Similarly, choroideremia is not known to affect blood vessels elsewhere in the body, and it is therefore likely that choroidal atrophy is occurring as a secondary phenomenon in response to loss of the overlying retinal pigment epithelium. In other retinal conditions, the choroid undergoes progressive atrophy many years after subretinal surgery if the pigment epithelium is damaged, leading to a gradual and focal unmasking of scleral autofluorescence, which is similar to the progression of choroideremia (MacLaren et al. 2005). Despite this, a slow primary degeneration of the choroid cannot be excluded completely.

Taken together, the data above indicate that it is logical to propose that gene therapy for choroideremia should use viral vectors that definitively target both rod photoreceptors and RPE cells. There is not strong evidence to propose using a vector that targets choroidal tissue, and transducing cones photoreceptor cells should possibly be avoided. In this respect AAV is again a good choice, as it can effectively target and transfer DNA to (transduce) the specific cell types and tissues that need to be treated. There are many different AAV subtypes, each with slightly different DNA sequences and capsid proteins on their outer shell (serotypes). These serotypes have different cellular tropism; they preferentially target specific cell types within a given host species. Many AAV vectors target neurons effectively but AAV serotype 2 has been shown to transduce photoreceptors and the RPE after subretinal injection in non-human primates (Bennett et al. 1999; Jacobson et al. 2006a). AAV2 appears to predominantly target rods, rather than cones (Bennett et al. 1999), which may be better from a safety perspective, but avoiding cone transduction completely by using AAV2 cannot be guaranteed because there are many unknown factors operating in the degenerating retina. It seems unlikely that AAV2 will be able to bypass the combined barriers of the RPE and Bruch's membrane and tropism of AAV2 for the deeper vascular layers of the choroid has been relatively unexplored, but any possible transduction and treatment here could only be beneficial. As REP1 is normally ubiquitously expressed, the unlikely event of a more widespread transduction pattern of the gene therapy virus might not be considered a major cause for concern, even in cells and tissue outside the eye.

In further support of the use of AAV2, there is extensive safety data in primates (Jacobson et al. 2006a), and recent gene therapy clinical trials for Leber congenital amaurosis type 2 (LCA2) using AAV2-RPE65 show subretinal administration does not cause significant immunogenicity, inflammation or toxicity (Bainbridge et al. 2008; Maguire et al. 2008; Hauswirth et al. 2008). Data from dog models of LCA2 treated with AAV2-RPE65 show that they have maintained vision without reduction for several years and even over a decade in some cases (Bennicelli et al. 2008; Cideciyan et al. 2013). In the human trials, visual gains following gene transfer are sustained for at least 3 years (Jacobson et al. 2012; Testa et al. 2013; Cideciyan et al. 2013).

In summary, AAV2 displays tropism for the correct cell types, is capable of packaging the full REP1 coding sequence and has been shown to be safe and effective for up to 3 years in ocular gene therapy trials for a different inherited eye disease (namely, LCA2). Thus, AAV2 was selected for use in a REP1-replacement gene therapy strategy for choroideremia and was such a compelling choice; it appeared futile to undertake a detailed consideration of the use of other types of virus, such as lentiviruses and adenoviruses.

3.3.3 Designing an Efficient AAV2-REP1 Expression Cassette (the Construct)

As REP1 is expressed ubiquitously, there would be little worth in identifying its 5′ upstream promoter sequence to drive regulated transgene expression. We chose instead to use a well-characterised ubiquitous promoter, capable of driving sustained, high levels of expression. For this purpose, a hybrid of the human cytomegalovirus (CMV) upstream enhancer with the chicken beta-actin promoter (usually termed CAG) has been used extensively in preclinical studies by a large number of groups. The original CBA promoter construct was generated in Japan (Niwa et al. 1991; Miyazaki et al. 1989) and used successfully in AAV in vivo first by Mark Sands in the USA (Daly et al. 1999). It was subsequently shown to be highly effective in the brain (Klein et al. 2000). A later study showed that an AAV vector with the CAG promoter resulted in 9.5-fold higher expression after portal vein injection than an AAV vector with the EF1alpha promoter and 137-fold higher expression than an AAV vector with the CMV promoter/enhancer (Xu et al. 2001). CBA-based promoters show highly effective transduction in retinal gene therapy clinical trials (Maguire et al. 2008; Hauswirth et al. 2008) and appear to give sustained expression for over a decade in dogs (Bennicelli et al. 2008; Cideciyan et al. 2013) and at least 3 years in humans (Jacobson et al. 2012; Testa et al. 2013; Cideciyan et al. 2013). Although the lifelong effects in humans will not be known for some time, these data suggest that expression from the CAG promoter in the AAV2 vector is sustained and early loss of therapeutic transgene expression though mechanism of gene silencing, such as methylation of the promoter DNA, is not a significant issue.

Other sequences in the transgene expression cassette were also used to generate robust expression of the therapeutic gene. Both in vitro and in vivo, AAV transgene expression has been shown to be enhanced by the inclusion of a woodchuck hepatitis virus post-transcriptional regulatory element (WPRE) downstream of the gene coding sequence (Paterna et al. 2000; Klein et al. 2002; Loeb et al. 1999). Although this element has not been used in previous retinal gene therapy trials, the same WPRE sequence was approved by the US Food and Drug Administration (FDA) for use in AAV2-GAD gene therapy trials in Parkinson's disease. This did not lead to any severe adverse events and there was even evidence of functional improvement at one year (Kaplitt et al. 2007). Notably, this WPRE sequence has been modified to ablate the translation initiation site of the viral X antigen, which has previously been proposed possibly to increase tumour susceptibility in the liver of mice receiving large doses (Flajolet et al. 1998). The WPRE, however, has not been observed to cause any similar problems in a number of laboratory studies since, and it is notable that Glybera®, the only approved gene therapy product to date, also includes a WPRE in the AAV expression cassette. Gene expression can also be enhanced by the specific polyadenylation (polyA) signal sequence used. The polyA sequence of bovine growth hormone (BGH) we opted for can yield three times higher expression levels than other polyA sequences such as SV40 and human collagen polyA, and this increase has been shown to be largely independent of the type of upstream promoter or transgene (Pfarr et al. 1986). A vital component of the cassette is the cDNA sequence encoding human REP1, which has previously been fully cloned and characterised (Cremers et al. 1990; van Bokhoven et al. 1994).

Finally, AAV expression cassettes must be flanked by identical inverted terminal repeat (ITR) sequences. These are the only remaining part of the genome of wild-type AAV used in the vector and are important in packaging the single-stranded DNA into virions and also in somehow protecting and maintaining the unpackaged DNA in an episomal state in transduced cells. Most ITR sequences used for clinical trials (including ours) are derived from the genome of AAV2, regardless of which capsid serotype they are packaged into. Thus, the full annotation of the vector would be AAV2/2, to indicate that AAV2 ITRs have been used to package the expression cassette into the AAV2 serotype.

Overall, each AAV virion would contain a single-stranded DNA sequence of around 4.2 kb in length comprising of a cytomegalovirus enhancer/chicken beta-actin hybrid promoter (CAG), human REP1 cDNA, woodchuck hepatitis post-transcriptional regulatory element (WPRE) and bovine growth hormone polyadenylation sequence (BGH-polyA). This would all be flanked by inverted terminal repeat (ITR) sequences from the wild-type AAV2 genome.

AAV transgene expression level in our vector is maximised by a combination of an optimised promoter and polyA signal, along with the inclusion of WPRE sequence. Overall this allows a lower dose of AAV vector to be used to achieve the same therapeutic effect. This is likely to help minimise the immune response to viral proteins in patients. Although it might be argued that this could instead be achieved by using other AAV serotypes that produce more efficient expression, such as AAV8 (Lebherz et al. 2008), we decided that, in view of the long-term data on safety and sustained expression available for AAV2, it was preferential to optimise the expression cassette rather than switch capsids.

3.3.4 Preclinical Testing of the Vector

All preclinical work was conducted using AAV2-REP1 that had been packaged and purified to a research-grade standard, but was otherwise identical to the clinical-grade vector that could be used in a choroideremia clinical trial (Tolmachova et al. 2013). Testing of the gene therapy expression cassette also involved creation of a green fluorescent protein (GFP) reporter vector. In this reporter vector, the *REP1/Chm* cDNA was replaced with the coding sequence of GFP, but otherwise, the structure and sequence were identical. Subretinal injection of AAV2-GFP reporter vector in mice confirmed targeting of the transgene to RPE and a high level of expression in photoreceptors (Tolmachova et al. 2013). Moreover, in vitro explants of human retina in culture exposed to AAV2-GFP vector confirmed that the gene therapy expression cassette and capsid type were capable of transducing photoreceptors and driving a high level of transgene expression (Tolmachova et al. 2013).

The therapeutic AAV2-REP1 vector was able to produce the appropriate protein in cultured fibroblasts of choroideremia patients (as detected by Western blot). Crucially, by examining prenylation activity in these transduced cells, correct function of the REP1 transgene product could also be confirmed (Tolmachova et al. 2013). We did not detect impairment of retinal function (as assessed by electroretinography) after subretinal injection of AAV2-REP1 in wild-type mice, and thus, no obvious toxic effects are evident following overexpression of REP1 (Tolmachova et al. 2013). Naturally occurring, large animal models have also been used in the preclinical assessment of gene therapy for retinal disease such as LCA2 (Bennicelli et al. 2008; Cideciyan et al. 2013) and achromatopsia (Komaromy et al. 2010). Unfortunately, no such large animal model exists for choroideremia. There are also problems with the mouse model, for example, the genetic deletion of *Chm* causes embryonic lethality in hemizygous (*Chm^{null}/Y*) male mice (van den Hurk et al. 1997; Shi et al. 2004). However, carrier female mice (*Chm^{null/+}*) do exhibit progressive retinal degeneration and seem to be the most robust model of the phenotype in human-affected hemizygous males (van den Hurk et al. 1997; Tolmachova et al. 2006, 2010). Subretinal injection of AAV2-REP1 was used to treat *Chm^{null/+}* mice, and when assessed after several months and compared to paired sham control eyes, a dose-dependent improvement/preservation of retinal function was found (Tolmachova et al. 2013). Thus, using a range of techniques and experiments, the preclinical work confirmed the effectiveness and safety of the AAV2-REP1 gene therapy vector.

3.4   Description of the Trial

In the trial, patients with a genetic diagnosis of choroideremia undergo gene therapy using adeno-associated viral (AAV) vector encoding the REP1 protein of the CHM gene. As gene therapy treatment will be performed when retinal structure remains relatively intact (i.e. before major cell loss) and when 'good' foveal vision is still retained, surgical delivery of the virus presents a specific challenge. The vector is administered to the subretinal space by injection during vitrectomy surgery, and the potential risks are significant as the treatment involves detachment of the fovea in a patient with good visual acuity. In addition, although there is no preclinical evidence that REP1 is toxic, and it is present in virtually all nucleated cells in non-choroideremia patients, an unknown factor in the trial is the potential detrimental effect REP1 (over)expression might have on retinal cells, particularly functional photoreceptors. In addition, this is the first gene therapy trial for retinal degeneration that has specifically targeted photoreceptor cells (in trials for RPE65-LCA2, the RPE cells were the primary target). Hence, the primary objective of the study is to assess the safety and tolerability of the AAV2-REP1 vector. This is done by monitoring for evidence of ocular inflammation or detrimental effects to visual function in patients for 24 months after administration. Changes in the treated eye are compared to baseline measurements and to the fellow untreated eye.

In order to ensure that photoreceptor cells are not compromised, the trial involves an escalation of the vector dose from a low baseline level. The starting dose of AAV2 (10^{10} genome particles) is at the lower end of the range (10^{10}–10^{12}) that has been shown to be safe in current AAV2 ocular gene therapy trials (Bainbridge et al. 2008; Maguire et al. 2008; Hauswirth et al. 2008). Reactions to AAV capsid protein are therefore deemed unlikely because of this, even allowing for a large number of empty vector particles. However, the REP1 protein will be expressed against a null background, and there is a theoretical risk of immune reaction to a new protein and for this reason the initial vector doses tested is kept low. If no serious adverse effects or reactions are seen at the starting dose in the first group of six patients, then the dose of AAV2 will be increased up ten times higher (10^{11} genome particles) in the second group of six patients.

Although great consideration and planning must be used to ensure the surgery and vector are safe, ultimately, if no form of treatment is given, vision will eventually be lost due to the ongoing degeneration. The gene transfer to the photoreceptor and RPE cells might enable the cells to survive long term. Therefore, the secondary end point of the study is to identify any therapeutic benefit of subretinal injection of AAV2-REP1 vector. As choroideremia is a progressive disease, this would be evidenced by a slowing down of the visual function loss and retinal degeneration in the treated eye compared to the control eye, 24 months after gene delivery. A range of functional and anatomical ophthalmological tests and examinations will be used to assess this, but microperimetry, optical coherence tomography (OCT) scans and fundus autofluorescence imaging will be key.

3.4.1   The Approval Process

Clinical trials in the UK are regulated by the Medicines for Human Use (Clinical Trials) Regulations 2004 (SI 1031) as amended. These regulations implement Directive 2001/20/EC ('The Clinical Trials Directive'). According to the Clinical Trials Directive, clinical trials of medicinal products in human subjects require authorisation by the competent authority and a favourable opinion by an ethics committee. In the UK, for ethical approval of a gene therapy clinical trial, you must apply to the UK Department of Health Gene Therapy Advisory Committee (GTAC). GTAC is the UK National Research Ethics Committee (REC) for gene therapy clinical research according to regulation 14(5) of the Medicines for Human Use (Clinical Trials) Regulations 2004. The Medicines and Healthcare Products Regulatory Agency (MHRA) is the competent authority for determining clinical trial authorisation in the UK. The trial protocol and preclinical safety and efficacy data were

submitted and presented to these bodies over the course of several months. The choroideremia trial was reviewed first by GTAC. It received a favourable opinion (under the reference GTAC0171) and so the application could be submitted to MHRA. This application was approved and the trial was also registered with the European Union Drug Regulating Authorities Clinical Trials under the reference EudraCT 2009-014617-27. Local ethics committees for each of four participating sites (Oxford Eye Hospital, Moorfields Eye Hospital, Manchester Royal Eye Hospital and the Eye Department of Southampton General Hospital) also approved the study. Major funding was obtained from the Health Innovation Challenge Fund, a parallel funding partnership between the Wellcome Trust and the UK Department of Health, and the trial was registered at ClinicalTrials.gov (identifier: NCT01461213).

Although there has likely never been an approval process that is entirely without its problems, the application for choroideremia gene therapy was not notably gruelling. Overall the regulators took a pragmatic view and accepted that the safety profile of AAV gene therapy in humans was already quite well established and specifically that AAV2 had been administered to the human eye with no significant harm (Hauswirth et al. 2008; Bainbridge et al. 2008; Maguire et al. 2008). The regulators did not insist on our repeating costly and time-consuming experiments for AAV-REP1, such as vector biodistribution studies in non-human primates, which would not be relevant anyway in view of the choroidal atrophy in the trial participants. The regulator took the enlightened view that the preclinical data from the mouse model and from the expression and functional assays in patient cells in vitro were sufficient evidence to proceed to a human trial and did not insist on the use of a large animal model (which does not currently exist for choroideremia).

Indeed, at this time, the largest barrier to gene therapy research in the UK is not the trial approval process. In fact, it is the ever-increasing cost of conducting the animal research necessary to produce high-quality preclinical data that may be holding back faster progress. We do not doubt that the exorbitant housing and husbandry costs for laboratory mice combined with an inordinate amount of time needed to navigate the (sometimes irrational and highly mutable) local and national regulations may make the West an increasingly uncompetitive global location to conduct biomedical research.

3.4.2 The Manufacturing

We chose to use the biotechnology company GeneDetect to produce research-grade AAV that could be used in preclinical testing (Tolmachova et al. 2013). Through this company's licensing agreements and links with Professor Matthew During, we were able from the outset to work with an AAV2 expression cassette and production protocols that had previously been scaled up to current Good Manufacturing Practice (cGMP), approved by the US Food and Drug Administration (FDA) and used safely in patients in another gene therapy trial (Kaplitt et al. 2007). Therefore, all our preclinical work was conducted using an AAV2 vector expressing REP1 that has been packaged and purified by GeneDetect to a research-grade standard, but is otherwise identical to the GMP-grade vector that would be used in the choroideremia clinical trial. This integration allowed us to translate safely from the laboratory to a clinical trial, when moving from research grade to GMP for AAV manufacture. The AAV2-REP1 vector for clinical use was made to cGMP and consistent with the FDA's 'Guidance for Industry – cGMP for Phase 1 Investigational Drugs', at the Clinical Manufacturing Facility of the Nationwide Children's Hospital (NCH), Columbus, Ohio. A qualified person (QP) acting on behalf of the UK MHRA inspected the GMP facility at NCH in advance, to ensure that protocols were aligned with both FDA and UK MHRA recommended standards. In-process, bulk intermediate and final drug product release testing met all predetermined testing specifications in accordance to guidance from the MHRA. Importation, storage and QP release were organised by the MHRA-approved Clinical Biomanufacturing Facility at the University of Oxford.

3.4.3 Enrolment and the First Patients

The characteristic appearance of the fundus was used to first identify choroideremia clinically, but to be included in the study, patients need to have genetic testing at a National Health Service accredited laboratory and molecular diagnosis of a pathogenic, null mutation in the CHM gene confirmed, to avoid the inclusion of patients with other diseases with a similar appearance (e.g. gyrate atrophy, Oliver-McFarlane syndrome, progressive bifocal chorioretinal atrophy (PBCRA)). Healthy volunteers are not appropriate and were not eligible for inclusion.

Patients need to have symmetrical disease with no other co-pathologies (e.g. no macular hole) as the fellow eye is used as a control. Best corrected visual acuity (BCVA) has to be good enough to read letters on a standard ETDRS (early treatment for diabetic retinopathy study) vision chart, and patient have to be able to perform reliable microperimetry. No upper limit of visual acuity is set, the aim being to treat patients with 6/6 vision, if reliable and consistent defects in microperimetry can be identified within the macular area. The decision about which eye to treat is made on clinical grounds and considering patient preference. So far, the most affected/worst eye has been chosen for treatment in the majority of cases. We decided that, as the disease is X-linked, only male patients would be included in the study. Although choroideremia carrier females may have visual impairment, the rate of progression is generally much slower and more variable than in affected males. Consequently, it would be difficult to determine the secondary trial end point in terms of proven efficacy in female patients. A full list of inclusion criteria can be found in Table 3.1.

Potential patients were identified and enrolled from the study centres (Oxford Eye Hospital, Moorfields Eye Hospital, Manchester Royal Eye Hospital and the Eye Department of Southampton General Hospital). Patient selection was agreed between the study clinical investigators who reviewed scans, molecular diagnoses and clinical data. The general principle was to enrol patients during the most active stages of the disease, when

Table 3.1 Inclusion and exclusion criteria used when enrolling participants in the gene therapy trial for choroideremia

Inclusion criteria
Participant is willing and able to give informed consent for participation in the study. Male aged 18 years or above
Diagnosed with choroideremia and in good health
Active disease with scanning laser ophthalmoscope (SLO) changes visible within the macula region
Willing to allow his or her family doctor and ophthalmology consultant, if appropriate, to be notified of participation in the study
Vision at least 6/60 or better in the study eye
Exclusion criteria (the participant may not enter the study if ANY of the following apply)
Female and child participants (under the age of 18)
Men unwilling to use barrier contraception methods, if relevant
Previous history of retinal surgery or ocular inflammatory disease (uveitis)
Grossly asymmetrical disease or other ocular morbidity which might confound use of the fellow eye as a long-term control
Any other significant disease or disorder which, in the opinion of the investigator, may either put the participants at risk because of participation in the study or may influence the result of the study, or the participant's ability to participate in the study. This would include not taking or having a contraindication to oral prednisolone, such as a history of gastric ulcer or significant side effects
Participants who have participated in another research study involving an investigational product in the past 12 weeks

changes in retinal appearance are taking place in the posterior pole of the eye. This region can be subjected to detailed image analysis using the scanning laser ophthalmoscope (SLO), visual field testing and multifocal electroretinogram (ERG) analysis (see below for more information on the tests). Hence, patients with very early disease and minimal visible changes would not be enrolled. Effectively this excludes children in the early trials, and it may not be justifiable in view of the risks of retinal damage from potential complications in an early intervention. As a consequence, the consent and information brochures are set up for adult subjects accordingly, and to be eligible for the study, patients had to be adults (18 years and older). All procedures followed were in accordance with the ethical standards of the responsible committee on human experimentation (institutional and national) and with the Helsinki Declaration of 1975, as revised in 2000. Informed consent was obtained from all patients for being included in the study.

3.4.4 The Tests

The primary outcome measure of the trial is best corrected visual acuity (BCVA). At the early stages after treatment, we look for detrimental effects on visual function by assessing the patient's ability to read letters on a standard ETDRS (early treatment for diabetic retinopathy study) vision chart using each eye. Patients generally maintain good visual acuity until the degeneration encroaches on the fovea, so this outcome measure will not be relevant in assessing treatment efficacy in most cases. BCVA testing will be part of the clinical examination which will also include fundoscopy, to monitor for signs of inflammation, cataract or retinal detachment.

There are seven further assessments of vision performed at various timepoints during the study as outlined in Table 3.2. These are comprised of three anatomical assessments (fundus photography, autofluorescence and OCT scan) and four functional tests (Humphrey 30–2 perimetry, Goldman visual field, microperimetry and multifocal ERG). These tests will be used as secondary outcome measures in assessing safety but will also be important in assessing treatment efficacy. Although it is not expected that any anatomical parameter will show an improvement posttreatment compared to baseline, it is possible that there will be some recovery and restoration of vision when measured by the functional tests (retinal cells may be reversibly compromised before they undergo cell death). These gains might be detected by microperimetry testing, as

Table 3.2 Schedule of visual test during and after the trial. Testing to the left of the thickened vertical line is part of the trial and annual testing represents normal UK National Health Service (NHS) care

Clinical Tests/month:	Baseline	1	6	12	24	Annual
1. Clinical examination[a]	✔	✔	✔	✔	✔	✔
2. Fundus photography	✔	✔	✔	✔	✔	✔
3. Fundus autofluorescence	✔	✔	✔	✔	✔	✔
4. Spectral domain OCT	✔	✔	✔	✔	✔	✔
5. Humphrey 30-2 perimetry	✔			✔	✔	✔
6. Goldmann visual field	✔			✔	✔	✔
7. Nidek MP1 microperimetry	✔			✔	✔	✔
8. Multifocal ERG	✔			✔	✔	✔

[a]Routine clinical examination will also take place in Oxford the day after surgery and at 1–2 weeks, in order to check for the known complications of vitrectomy, such as retinal detachment and raised intraocular pressure. Although no specific retinal investigations will take place at these initial post-operative visits, it will provide an opportunity to screen for any serious adverse event/reaction that might trigger stopping rules

significant deficits in parafoveal retinal sensitivity have previously been seen in even in the early stages of choroideremia (Jacobson et al. 2006b). The trial also includes some test of systemic immunology. These represent part of the general safety monitoring of the patient and may provide possible background data for future retreatment of the fellow eye, but are not included as trial end points. After formal trial testing, patients will continue to be monitored at one of the four referring centres as part of their normal NHS care. Annual checks continue, with additional tests performed at the discretion of the managing clinician. This monitoring includes a full history and physical examination to detect any possible malignancies, and any emerging safety concerns would be referred directly to the MHRA.

3.4.5 The Results

The study started in October 2012 and is ongoing. So far we have assessed and reported interim results for the first six patients, up to 6 months after treatment (Maclaren et al. 2014). These patients were recruited with a range of baseline visual acuities. Four patients with near-normal visual acuity at baseline experienced a transient drop in vision after treatment, which soon recovered without any signs of significant detrimental effects of the surgery or vector administration at 6 months after treatment. These results are encouraging from a safety perspective, but more remarkably, and in truth unexpectedly, two patients with advanced choroideremia and reduced baseline acuity actually had substantial gains in visual acuity 6 months after subretinal administration of the AAV-REP1. In the cohort as a whole, there was also an improvement in maximal retinal sensitivity in the eyes treated with AAV-REP1 (measured using microperimetry), despite detachment of the macula, which is usually associated with a reduction in retinal sensitivity. These improvements have been sustained in the 2 years since the single treatment, in the patients that have been followed up that long (MacLaren et al. 2014 – data presented at ARVO). Scepticism in science is healthy; we admit these gains may at first seem unbelievable and it is true that gene therapy cannot restore function from cells that have already been lost. However, it is very likely that improvement comes from a population of cells that are not yet dead but are reversibly compromised and therefore capable of benefiting from gene replacement.

Some care and caution is needed with the functional tests as they are all ultimately subjective (relying on the patient response) and the treatment is open label (both the patients and the clinical team know which eye is the injected), potentially exposing the trial to criticism of (intentional and unintentional) bias. There are some strong arguments against this, including the correlation of microperimetry gains with the dose of vector applied per mm^2 of surviving retinal pigment epithelium (RPE)-retina measured at baseline (Maclaren et al. 2014), which is something that it would be hard for those involved to prejudice. However, over longer-term follow-up, it will be interesting to see if differences evolve between treated and untreated eyes in the more objective anatomical/structural measurements such as OCT scan thickness and fundus autofluorescence area. This would indicate that disease progression and retinal degeneration have been halted or significantly slowed due to AAV-REP1 and might convince any remaining sceptics and critics. This will be apparent in due course, and we wait, impatiently, for the answer along with others.

The results so far have been greeted with cautious optimism (Huckfeldt and Bennett 2014), and it has been recognised that an important wider implication of the study is that good visual acuity can recover to baseline levels despite detachment of the fovea as part of the surgical procedure, which potential opens up a range of inherited retinal disease for treatment with gene therapy (Scholl and Sahel 2014).

3.5 Future Plans

Early results on the safety and efficacy of AAV2-REP1 gene therapy for choroideremia are very encouraging (Maclaren et al. 2014). We will be continuing with the current study while working to set up follow-on clinical trials using the same vector at the efficacious dose. We hope that further results and future studies continue to support the use of gene therapy in choroideremia and, if so, would like to see this become a 'routine' treatment.

Indeed, 'NightstaRx Limited' has been set up to aid the transition of clinical trial gene therapies for retinal dystrophies, such as this, into the domain of a marketable treatment option. Nightstar is a newly formed spin-out company from the University of Oxford and its research commercialisation arm, Isis Innovation, and is to receive a £12 million investment from Syncona, an independent subsidary of the Wellcome Trust. It is anticipated that an early programme of work for the company will be assisting in the clinical development of gene therapy for choroideremia, including the manufacture of AAV-REP1 to the stringent requirements needed for regulatory approval as a medical product and treatment. As the Wellcome Trust is ultimately a charitable organisation, the goal is not to make a large return on the investment and/or for the work to financially benefit those involved. It is expected, rather, that the large capital investment will yield faster and more efficient results in the commercial and corporate environment of a spin-out biopharmaceutical company than if development continues in a purely academic setting. Choroideremia patients will ultimately benefit from this approach, as it is designed to expedite their access to the therapy.

Acknowledgements The authors' work is supported by the NIHR Biomedical Research Centres at the Oxford University Hospitals and Moorfields Eye Hospital NHS Trusts. Additional funding is provided by the Health Foundation, Fight for Sight, the Lanvern Foundation, the Special Trustees of Moorfields Eye Hospital and the Royal College of Surgeons of Edinburgh. The CHM gene therapy clinical trial is funded by the Health Innovation Challenge Fund, a parallel funding partnership between the Wellcome Trust and the UK Department of Health.

Compliance with Ethical Requirements Where the authors' own research is presented and described in this chapter, we can confirm the following:
- For research involving humans: All procedures followed were in accordance with the ethical standards of the responsible committee on human experimentation (institutional and national) and with the Helsinki Declaration of 1975, as revised in 2000 (5). Informed consent was obtained from all patients for being included in the study.
- For research involving animals: All institutional and national guidelines for the care and use of laboratory animals were followed.

The authors declare the following conflicts of interest:

Author REM is a named coinventor on UK patent application 1103062.4, filed on Feb 22, 2011, and owned by the University of Oxford. Author REM is also a Director of NightstaRx (Welcome Trust Building, 215 Euston Road, London, UK), a choroideremia gene therapy company established by the University of Oxford and funded by the Wellcome Trust.

Author ARB and Author MG declare that they have no conflict of interest.

References

Bainbridge JW, Smith AJ, Barker SS, Robbie S, Henderson R, Balaggan K, Viswanathan A, Holder GE, Stockman A, Tyler N, Petersen-Jones S, Bhattacharya SS, Thrasher AJ, Fitzke FW, Carter BJ, Rubin GS, Moore AT, Ali RR (2008) Effect of gene therapy on visual function in Leber's congenital amaurosis. N Engl J Med 358(21):2231–2239. doi:10.1056/NEJMoa0802268

Bennett J, Maguire AM, Cideciyan AV, Schnell M, Glover E, Anand V, Aleman TS, Chirmule N, Gupta AR, Huang Y, Gao GP, Nyberg WC, Tazelaar J, Hughes J, Wilson JM, Jacobson SG (1999) Stable transgene expression in rod photoreceptors after recombinant adeno-associated virus-mediated gene transfer to monkey retina. Proc Natl Acad Sci U S A 96(17):9920–9925

Bennicelli J, Wright JF, Komaromy A, Jacobs JB, Hauck B, Zelenaia O, Mingozzi F, Hui D, Chung D, Rex TS, Wei Z, Qu G, Zhou S, Zeiss C, Arruda VR, Acland GM, Dell'Osso LF, High KA, Maguire AM, Bennett J (2008) Reversal of blindness in animal models of leber congenital amaurosis using optimized AAV2-mediated gene transfer. Mol Ther 16(3):458–465. doi:10.1038/sj.mt.6300389

Bonilha VL, Trzupek KM, Li Y, Francis PJ, Hollyfield JG, Rayborn ME, Smaoui N, Weleber RG (2008) Choroideremia: analysis of the retina from a female symptomatic carrier. Ophthalmic Genet 29(3):99–110. doi:10.1080/13816810802206499

Cideciyan AV, Jacobson SG, Beltran WA, Sumaroka A, Swider M, Iwabe S, Roman AJ, Olivares MB, Schwartz SB, Komaromy AM, Hauswirth WW, Aguirre GD (2013) Human retinal gene therapy for Leber congenital amaurosis shows advancing retinal degeneration despite enduring visual improvement. Proc Natl Acad Sci U S A 110(6):E517–E525. doi:10.1073/pnas.1218933110

Cremers FP, van de Pol DJ, van Kerkhoff LP, Wieringa B, Ropers HH (1990) Cloning of a gene that is rearranged in patients with choroideraemia. Nature 347(6294):674–677. doi:10.1038/347674a0

Cremers FP, Armstrong SA, Seabra MC, Brown MS, Goldstein JL (1994) REP-2, a Rab escort protein encoded by the choroideremia-like gene. J Biol Chem 269(3):2111–2117

Daly TM, Okuyama T, Vogler C, Haskins ME, Muzyczka N, Sands MS (1999) Neonatal intramuscular injection with recombinant adeno-associated virus results in prolonged beta-glucuronidase expression in situ and correction of liver pathology in mucopolysaccharidosis type VII mice. Hum Gene Ther 10(1):85–94. doi:10.1089/10430349950019219

Flajolet M, Tiollais P, Buendia MA, Fourel G (1998) Woodchuck hepatitis virus enhancer I and enhancer II are both involved in N-myc2 activation in woodchuck liver tumors. J Virol 72(7):6175–6180

Flannery JG, Bird AC, Farber DB, Weleber RG, Bok D (1990) A histopathologic study of a choroideremia carrier. Invest Ophthalmol Vis Sci 31(2):229–236

Hauswirth WW, Aleman TS, Kaushal S, Cideciyan AV, Schwartz SB, Wang L, Conlon TJ, Boye SL, Flotte TR, Byrne BJ, Jacobson SG (2008) Treatment of leber congenital amaurosis due to RPE65 mutations by ocular subretinal injection of adeno-associated virus gene vector: short-term results of a phase I trial. Hum Gene Ther 19(10):979–990. doi:10.1089/hum.2008.107

Huckfeldt RM, Bennett J (2014) Promising first steps in gene therapy for choroideremia. Hum Gene Ther 25(2):96–97. doi:10.1089/hum.2014.2503

Jacobson SG, Boye SL, Aleman TS, Conlon TJ, Zeiss CJ, Roman AJ, Cideciyan AV, Schwartz SB, Komaromy AM, Doobrajh M, Cheung AY, Sumaroka A, Pearce-Kelling SE, Aguirre GD, Kaushal S, Maguire AM, Flotte TR, Hauswirth WW (2006a) Safety in nonhuman primates of ocular AAV2-RPE65, a candidate treatment for blindness in Leber congenital amaurosis. Hum Gene Ther 17(8):845–858. doi:10.1089/hum.2006.17.845

Jacobson SG, Cideciyan AV, Sumaroka A, Aleman TS, Schwartz SB, Windsor EA, Roman AJ, Stone EM, MacDonald IM (2006b) Remodeling of the human retina in choroideremia: rab escort protein 1 (REP-1) mutations. Invest Ophthalmol Vis Sci 47(9):4113–4120. doi:10.1167/iovs.06-0424

Jacobson SG, Cideciyan AV, Ratnakaram R, Heon E, Schwartz SB, Roman AJ, Peden MC, Aleman TS, Boye SL, Sumaroka A, Conlon TJ, Calcedo R, Pang JJ, Erger KE, Olivares MB, Mullins CL, Swider M, Kaushal S, Feuer WJ, Iannaccone A, Fishman GA, Stone EM, Byrne BJ, Hauswirth WW (2012) Gene therapy for leber congenital amaurosis caused by RPE65 mutations: safety and efficacy in 15 children and adults followed up to 3 years. Arch Ophthalmol 130(1):9–24. doi:10.1001/archophthalmol.2011.298

Kaplitt MG, Feigin A, Tang C, Fitzsimons HL, Mattis P, Lawlor PA, Bland RJ, Young D, Strybing K, Eidelberg D, During MJ (2007) Safety and tolerability of gene therapy with an adeno-associated virus (AAV) borne GAD gene for Parkinson's disease: an open label, phase I trial. Lancet 369(9579):2097–2105. doi:10.1016/S0140-6736(07)60982-9

Klein RL, Mandel RJ, Muzyczka N (2000) Adeno-associated virus vector-mediated gene transfer to somatic cells in the central nervous system. Adv Virus Res 55:507–528

Klein RL, Hamby ME, Gong Y, Hirko AC, Wang S, Hughes JA, King MA, Meyer EM (2002) Dose and promoter effects of adeno-associated viral vector for green fluorescent protein expression in the rat brain. Exp Neurol 176(1):66–74

Komaromy AM, Alexander JJ, Rowlan JS, Garcia MM, Chiodo VA, Kaya A, Tanaka JC, Acland GM, Hauswirth WW, Aguirre GD (2010) Gene therapy rescues cone function in congenital achromatopsia. Hum Mol Genet 19(13):2581–2593. doi:10.1093/hmg/ddq136

Larijani B, Hume AN, Tarafder AK, Seabra MC (2003) Multiple factors contribute to inefficient prenylation of Rab27a in Rab prenylation diseases. J Biol Chem 278(47):46798–46804. doi:10.1074/jbc.M307799200

Lebherz C, Maguire A, Tang W, Bennett J, Wilson JM (2008) Novel AAV serotypes for improved ocular gene transfer. J Gene Med 10(4):375–382. doi:10.1002/jgm.1126

Loeb JE, Cordier WS, Harris ME, Weitzman MD, Hope TJ (1999) Enhanced expression of transgenes from adeno-associated virus vectors with the woodchuck hepatitis virus posttranscriptional regulatory element: implications for gene therapy. Hum Gene Ther 10(14):2295–2305. doi:10.1089/10430349950016942

MacDonald IM, Russell L, Chan CC (2009) Choroideremia: new findings from ocular pathology and review of recent literature. Surv Ophthalmol 54(3):401–407. doi:10.1016/j.survophthal.2009.02.008

MacLaren RE, Bird AC, Sathia PJ, Aylward GW (2005) Long-term results of submacular surgery combined with macular translocation of the retinal pigment epithelium in neovascular age-related macular degeneration. Ophthalmology 112(12):2081–2087. doi:10.1016/j.ophtha.2005.06.029

Maclaren RE, Groppe M, Barnard AR, Cottriall CL, Tolmachova T, Seymour L, Clark KR, During MJ, Cremers FP, Black GC, Lotery AJ, Downes SM, Webster AR, Seabra MC (2014) Retinal gene therapy in patients with choroideremia: initial findings from a phase 1/2 clinical trial. Lancet. doi:10.1016/S0140-6736(13)62117-0

Maguire AM, Simonelli F, Pierce EA, Pugh EN Jr, Mingozzi F, Bennicelli J, Banfi S, Marshall KA, Testa F, Surace EM, Rossi S, Lyubarsky A, Arruda VR, Konkle B, Stone E, Sun J, Jacobs J, Dell'Osso L, Hertle R, Ma JX, Redmond TM, Zhu X, Hauck B, Zelenaia O, Shindler KS, Maguire MG, Wright JF, Volpe NJ, McDonnell JW, Auricchio A, High KA, Bennett J (2008) Safety and efficacy of gene transfer for Leber's congenital amaurosis. N Engl J Med 358(21):2240–2248. doi:10.1056/NEJMoa0802315

Mauthner L (1872) Ophthalmologische Mittheilungen: 2. Ein Fall von Chorioidemie. In: Berichte des naturwissenschaftlichen-medizinischen Verein Innsbruck, vol 2. Medical and Scientific Association Innsbruck, Innsbruck: Austria; pp 191–197

Merry DE, Janne PA, Landers JE, Lewis RA, Nussbaum RL (1992) Isolation of a candidate gene for choroideremia. Proc Natl Acad Sci U S A 89(6):2135–2139

Miyazaki J, Takaki S, Araki K, Tashiro F, Tominaga A, Takatsu K, Yamamura K (1989) Expression vector system based on the chicken beta-actin promoter directs efficient production of interleukin-5. Gene 79(2):269–277

Myers T (2006) Mosby's dictionary of medicine, nursing & health professions, 7th edn. Mosby Elsevier, St. Louis/London

Niwa H, Yamamura K, Miyazaki J (1991) Efficient selection for high-expression transfectants with a novel eukaryotic vector. Gene 108(2):193–199

Paterna JC, Moccetti T, Mura A, Feldon J, Bueler H (2000) Influence of promoter and WHV posttranscriptional regulatory element on AAV-mediated transgene expression in the rat brain. Gene Ther 7(15):1304–1311. doi:10.1038/sj.gt.3301221

Pfarr DS, Rieser LA, Woychik RP, Rottman FM, Rosenberg M, Reff ME (1986) Differential effects of polyadenylation regions on gene expression in mammalian cells. DNA 5(2):115–122

Pylypenko O, Rak A, Reents R, Niculae A, Sidorovitch V, Cioaca MD, Bessolitsyna E, Thoma NH, Waldmann H, Schlichting I, Goody RS, Alexandrov K (2003) Structure of Rab escort protein-1 in complex with Rab geranylgeranyltransferase. Mol Cell 11(2):483–494

Reese BE, Harvey AR, Tan SS (1995) Radial and tangential dispersion patterns in the mouse retina are cell-class specific. Proc Natl Acad Sci U S A 92(7):2494–2498

Sankila EM, Tolvanen R, van den Hurk JA, Cremers FP, de la Chapelle A (1992) Aberrant splicing of the CHM gene is a significant cause of choroideremia. Nat Genet 1(2):109–113. doi:10.1038/ng0592-109

Scholl HP, Sahel JA (2014) Gene therapy arrives at the macula. Lancet 383(9923):1105–1107. doi:10.1016/S0140-6736(14)60033-7

Seabra MC, Brown MS, Slaughter CA, Sudhof TC, Goldstein JL (1992a) Purification of component A of Rab geranylgeranyl transferase: possible identity with the choroideremia gene product. Cell 70(6):1049–1057

Seabra MC, Goldstein JL, Sudhof TC, Brown MS (1992b) Rab geranylgeranyl transferase. A multisubunit enzyme that prenylates GTP-binding proteins terminating in Cys-X-Cys or Cys-Cys. J Biol Chem 267(20):14497–14503

Seabra MC, Brown MS, Goldstein JL (1993) Retinal degeneration in choroideremia: deficiency of rab geranylgeranyl transferase. Science 259(5093):377–381

Seabra MC, Ho YK, Anant JS (1995) Deficient geranylgeranylation of Ram/Rab27 in choroideremia. J Biol Chem 270(41):24420–24427

Shi W, van den Hurk JA, Alamo-Bethencourt V, Mayer W, Winkens HJ, Ropers HH, Cremers FP, Fundele R (2004) Choroideremia gene product affects trophoblast development and vascularization in mouse extra-embryonic tissues. Dev Biol 272(1):53–65. doi:10.1016/j.ydbio.2004.04.016

Syed N, Smith JE, John SK, Seabra MC, Aguirre GD, Milam AH (2001) Evaluation of retinal photoreceptors and pigment epithelium in a female carrier of choroideremia. Ophthalmology 108(4):711–720

Testa F, Maguire AM, Rossi S, Pierce EA, Melillo P, Marshall K, Banfi S, Surace EM, Sun J, Acerra C, Wright JF, Wellman J, High KA, Auricchio A, Bennett J, Simonelli F (2013) Three-year follow-up after unilateral subretinal delivery of adeno-associated virus in patients with Leber congenital Amaurosis type 2. Ophthalmology 120(6):1283–1291. doi:10.1016/j.ophtha.2012.11.048

Tolmachova T, Ramalho JS, Anant JS, Schultz RA, Huxley CM, Seabra MC (1999) Cloning, mapping and characterization of the human RAB27A gene. Gene 239(1):109–116

Tolmachova T, Anders R, Abrink M, Bugeon L, Dallman MJ, Futter CE, Ramalho JS, Tonagel F, Tanimoto N, Seeliger MW, Huxley C, Seabra MC (2006) Independent degeneration of photoreceptors and retinal pigment epithelium in conditional knockout mouse models of choroideremia. J Clin Invest 116(2):386–394. doi:10.1172/JCI26617

Tolmachova T, Wavre-Shapton ST, Barnard AR, MacLaren RE, Futter CE, Seabra MC (2010) Retinal pigment epithelium defects accelerate photoreceptor degeneration in cell type-specific knockout mouse models of choroideremia. Invest Ophthalmol Vis Sci 51(10):4913–4920. doi:10.1167/iovs.09-4892

Tolmachova T, Tolmachov OE, Barnard AR, de Silva SR, Lipinski DM, Walker NJ, Maclaren RE, Seabra MC (2013) Functional expression of Rab escort protein 1 following AAV2-mediated gene delivery in the retina of choroideremia mice and human cells ex vivo. J Mol Med 91(7):825–837. doi:10.1007/s00109-013-1006-4

van Bokhoven H, van den Hurk JA, Bogerd L, Philippe C, Gilgenkrantz S, de Jong P, Ropers HH, Cremers FP (1994) Cloning and characterization of the human choroideremia gene. Hum Mol Genet 3(7):1041–1046

van den Hurk JA, Hendriks W, van de Pol DJ, Oerlemans F, Jaissle G, Ruther K, Kohler K, Hartmann J, Zrenner E, van Bokhoven H, Wieringa B, Ropers HH, Cremers FP (1997) Mouse choroideremia gene mutation causes photoreceptor cell degeneration and is not transmitted through the female germline. Hum Mol Genet 6(6):851–858

Wu Z, Yang H, Colosi P (2010) Effect of genome size on AAV vector packaging. Mol Ther 18(1):80–86. doi:10.1038/mt.2009.255

Xu L, Daly T, Gao C, Flotte TR, Song S, Byrne BJ, Sands MS, Parker Ponder K (2001) CMV-beta-actin promoter directs higher expression from an adeno-associated viral vector in the liver than the cytomegalovirus or elongation factor 1 alpha promoter and results in therapeutic levels of human factor X in mice. Hum Gene Ther 12(5):563–573. doi:10.1089/104303401300042500

Gene Therapy for Dominantly Inherited Retinal Degeneration

4

Gwyneth Jane Farrar, Sophia Millington-Ward, Arpad Palfi, Naomi Chadderton, and Paul F. Kenna

4.1 Introduction

The genomics revolution over the past two decades has greatly enabled the elucidation of the genetic etiologies of many inherited conditions. Indeed significant progress has been made in defining the molecular pathogenesis of a group of hereditary eye diseases under the umbrella term retinal degenerations. This group of retinal dystrophies includes retinitis pigmentosa (RP), Leber congenital amaurosis (LCA), Usher syndrome (USH), congenital stationary night blindness (CSNB), vitelliform macular dystrophy, Stargardt disease, cone rod dystrophy, and age-related macular degeneration (AMD) among many others (see www.sph.uth.tmc.edu/retnet/ for details of disorders, causative genes, and mutations; Ayuso and Millan 2010). Typically, these hereditary disorders result in gradual loss of photoreceptor cells and compromised vision often leading to patients being registered as blind. The molecular pathogenesis of inherited ocular disorders primarily involving retinal cell layers other than the photoreceptor cell layer, for example, Leber hereditary optic neuropathy (LHON) involving

G.J. Farrar, PhD (✉) • S. Millington-Ward, PhD
A. Palfi, PhD • N. Chadderton, PhD
P.F. Kenna, MD, PhD, FRCSI
School of Genetics and Microbiology, Trinity College Dublin, Smurfit Institute of Genetics, Dublin, Ireland
e-mail: gjfarrar@tcd.ie; sophia@maths.tcd.ie; palfia@tcd.ie; chaddern@tcd.ie; pfkenna@tcd.ie

loss of retinal ganglion cells (RGC) in conjunction with optic atrophy, has also been elucidated (Wallace et al. 1988; Singh et al. 1989; Howell et al. 1991) as has dominant optic atrophy (DOA) primarily affecting the RGCs and optic nerve (Leanaers et al. 2012). Patterns of inheritance of retinal degenerations include autosomal recessive, autosomal dominant, X-linked, and mitochondrial inheritance. However, rare digenic forms of retinal dystrophies have also been characterized (Kajiwara et al. 1994; Fauser et al. 2003). The findings obtained from the large number of studies undertaken in the past few years have highlighted the immense genetic heterogeneity inherent in this group of conditions (Ferrari et al. 2011; Ratnapriya and Swaroop 2013). Thus, far approximately 250 genes have been implicated in inherited ocular disorders, approximately 70 of which are inherited in a dominant fashion, the topic of this chapter. Of note, many additional genes remain still to be identified.

RP is the most prevalent of the inherited retinal degenerations affecting approximately 1 in 3,000 people representing about a quarter of a million people in Europe (Ferrari et al. 2011). RP itself is characterized by extensive genetic heterogeneity with over 60 disease-causing genes implicated to date (www.sph.uth.edu/retnet/). Early studies in the field employed gene linkage technologies to localize disease-causing genes and resulted in the localization of the first X-linked RP (XlRP) and autosomal dominant RP (adRP) genes to X and 3q, respectively, about

E.P. Rakoczy (ed.), *Gene- and Cell-Based Treatment Strategies for the Eye*, Essentials in Ophthalmology, DOI 10.1007/978-3-662-45188-5_4, © Springer-Verlag Berlin Heidelberg 2015 three decades ago (Bhattacharya et al. 1984; McWilliam et al. 1989), with the subsequent characterization of RP2 and rhodopsin (*RHO*), respectively, as the causative genes (Dryja et al. 1990; Farrar et al. 1990; Schwahn et al. 1998). These initial findings were followed rapidly by many others exploiting approaches such as genetic linkage, positional cloning, homozygosity mapping, and sib pair analyses to identify genes implicated in inherited forms of retinal degeneration (Farrar et al. 1991; Kajiwara et al. 1991; Littink et al. 2012). An important feature of inherited retinopathies that has emerged from the large body of research undertaken to date is the enormous level of genetic heterogeneity inherent in these conditions, which has significant implications for their diagnosis, prognosis, and treatment; such heterogeneity pervades all genetic forms of retinal degenerations including dominant retinopathies.

Inherited retinal degenerations represent the most frequent cause of visual dysfunction in people of working age, and therefore, these conditions significantly influence quality of life over decades and economics. However, given the genetic heterogeneity inherent in inherited retinal disorders, genotypic characterization of disease-causing mutations, a prerequisite when designing gene therapies directed toward the primary mutation, is not trivial. Retinal microarrays have been developed to facilitate screening of known disease-causing mutations, for example, the retinal chip marketed by Asper Biotech (Asper Ophthalmic; www.asperophthalmics.coms). An alternative approach for rapid generation of high-throughput genotypic information is the use of next-generation sequencing (NGS) technologies based on massively parallel sequencing of millions of DNA fragments, technologies which are evolving to increase speed and capacity (Craig et al. 2008; Choi et al. 2009; Schweiger et al. 2009; Neveling et al. 2012; Audo et al. 2012; Glöckle et al. 2014). Indeed the relative merits of array-based mutation detection versus NGS for diagnosis of retinal disease have been compared, the latter providing higher rates of successful diagnosis and a more comprehensive probing of a wide array of mutations (Zaneveld et al. 2013).

NGS has been utilized to study retinal degeneration patient cohorts demonstrating a higher detection rate particularly in early onset disease (Shanks et al. 2013). Undoubtedly, NGS is an essential diagnostic tool that will play an increasingly important role in translating therapeutic development from the laboratory to the bedside. Exome and whole-genome sequencing will over the next few years move the dissection of the molecular genetics of these conditions to a new level.

While it is clear that there exists great diversity in the genetic pathogenesis of inherited retinal disorders and that future NGS studies undoubtedly will reveal additional genetic diversity, it is neverthelesss of interest to note that many of the disease mechanisms in operation in different Mendelian forms of retinal degenerations are common to each other and furthermore are mirrored in more prevalent multifactorial conditions such as age-related macular degeneration (AMD). AMD affects approximately 10 % of people over 65 years of age and results in a devastating and frequently rapid loss of vision.

Many common disease features are observed in AMD and RP including oxidative stress, mitochondrial dysfunction, and apoptotic cell death, among others. Hence, it is likely that advances in developing therapies for Mendelian disorders like RP may therefore be relevant to common disorders such as AMD and indeed such parallels have already been observed in, for example, oxidative stress and mitochondrial dysfunction and will be referred to in greater depth later in the chapter.

As noted above, the characterization of the molecular basis of inherited retinopathies will only serve to highlight further that disorders that are categorized together based on similarities in clinical presentation, when dissected at the molecular level, are extremely genetically heterogeneous involving multiple genes and indeed multiple disease-causing mutations within individual genes. The focus of this chapter is a subcategory of retinopathies, those inherited in an autosomal dominant fashion. However, even within this subcategory of disease, there exists significant intergenic and intragenic genetic

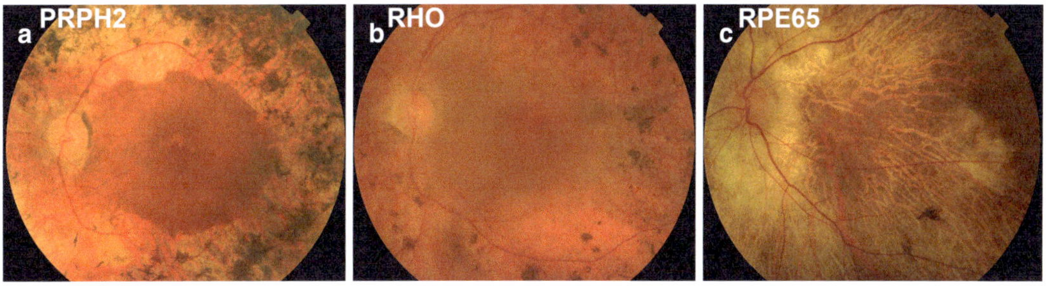

Fig. 4.1 Fundus photographs of adRP patients. Retinal fundus photographs from patients with three different genetic forms of adRP are presented; Ser212Gly *PRPH2* peripherin/*RDS* (**a**), Tyr178Cys *RHO* (**b**) and Asp477Gly *RPE65* (**c**)

heterogeneity, with over 70 genes implicated in dominant ocular disorders, 20 genes implicated in adRP (www.sph.uth.tmc.edu/RetNet), and more than 150 mutations identified to date solely within a single disease-causing gene, *RHO* (www.hgmd.cf.ac.uk/ac/index.php). Retinal fundus photographs of the three forms of adRP, *RHO*, peripherin/*RDS*, and *RPE65*-linked adRP are provided (Fig. 4.1a–c). Each of these causative genes was identified initially using large adRP pedigrees to undertake comprehensive linkage studies. Dominant inheritance typically results in families with multiple affected members thereby facilitating genetic localization of causative genes; the larger the family, the more robust the genetic linkage data obtained, where each family member contributes to a likelihood of the odds (Lod) score which describes the probability of linkage at a particular genomic location (Ott 1974). In Fig. 4.1c, the fundus of a patient with *RPE65*-adRP is presented. The RPE65 gene has been implicated in recessive forms of Leber congenital amaurosis (LCA); gene therapy trials for LCA have paved the way generally for the development of gene therapies for many inherited eye disorders as detailed below. It is recently that mutations in the RPE65 gene have also been implicated in a rare form of adRP as identified employing linkage and next-generation sequencing strategies (Bowne et al. 2011).

The significant level of genetic heterogeneity characteristic of many Mendelian and multifactorial ocular disorders represents a significant challenge when developing gene therapies for these diseases (Farrar et al. 2014). Various gene ther-

apy strategies that are being explored for the group of conditions termed dominantly inherited retinopathies will be outlined in this chapter. An overview of the approaches and associated technologies will be provided together with a summary of the preclinical data obtained thus far for some therapies, at times using examples of our research in Trinity College Dublin. Some of the technologies that emerged from Trinity College Dublin for dominantly inherited genetic disorders are now being developed in a company, Genable Technologies, also based in Dublin. While significant advances have been made in cell therapies and devices which could be applied to treatment of dominantly inherited ocular disorders, these fall outside the remit of this chapter.

4.2 Dominantly Inherited Retinopathies: Modes of Action

For X-linked recessive or autosomal recessive disorders involving the absence of wild-type protein, a rational therapeutic strategy is gene replacement. Indeed, results from clinical trials for Leber congenital amaurosis (LCA), a severe recessive retinopathy, initiated in 2008 (as Phase I/II trials) (Bainbridge et al. 2008, Maguire et al. 2008, Cideciyan et al. 2008) and currently progressing to a number of Phase III trials (reviewed in Mullard 2011), have elegantly demonstrated the principle of ocular gene therapy for recessively inherited retinopathies using a gene replacement approach, in this case employing the

RPE65 gene. Likewise, recent results from a clinical trial using adeno-associated virus (AAV)-mediated CHM gene replacement for X-linked recessive choroideremia have validated further the strategy (MacLaren et al. 2014). In contrast to recessive mutations where absence of the wild-type gene and encoded protein is universally implicated in disease etiology, the mode of action of dominant mutations can vary significantly between disorders. Mode of action will greatly influence which therapeutic strategy should be adopted, particularly for therapies directed toward amending the primary dominant mutation. Furthermore, frequently, the mode or modes of action may not be fully elucidated for any particular mutation thereby complicating the development of therapies and translation of such therapies into the clinic.

In principle, dominant disease pathologies may be orchestrated by the presence of the mutant protein, by reduced levels of wild-type protein, termed haploinsufficiency, or by a combination of both mechanisms together giving rise to the disease entities. For gene therapies targeted toward correcting the primary dominant mutation(s) driving disease processes, diverse strategies are being considered as briefly overviewed in this section and dealt with in depth later in the chapter. Some dominant conditions may require suppression of the mutant allele and encoded protein while maintaining expression of wild-type protein. However, frequently different mutations in the same gene can cause disease pathology. Indeed, for some dominant disorders, each family has almost a unique personalized mutation. If suppression is targeted toward the mutation site of the mutant allele, in principle, hundreds of therapies would be required each targeting a specific mutation. To overcome this, a mutation-independent strategy that corrects the primary genetic defect involving suppression and replacement has been explored (Millington-Ward et al. 1997, 2011; O'Reilly et al. 2007; Chadderton et al. 2009; Mao et al. 2012). This dual-component strategy involves suppression of both mutant and wild-type alleles in conjunction with provision of a modified replacement gene engineered to be refractory to suppression. Features of the genome

such as codon redundancy can be employed to engineer transcripts from replacement genes that are resistant to suppression due to the incorporation of nucleotide modifications over the target site for suppression (Millington-Ward et al. 1997, 2011). In principle, intragenic polymorphisms and/or modified untranslated regions (UTRs) could be employed (Millington-Ward et al. 1997) in replacement genes to achieve replacement genes refractory to suppression.

For any dominantly inherited disease, it is possible that gene replacement alone may provide some level of benefit. If haploinsufficiency is causative of at least some of the disease pathology, delivery of the wild-type allele to restore levels of the target protein toward those observed endogenously may provide benefit. In addition, even if haploinsufficiency is not causative of the dominant disease pathology, for some disorders, it may be that increasing the ratio of wild-type to mutant protein in favor of wild-type protein may modulate the dynamic of the disease process and provide a beneficial effect. Alternatively, for some conditions, a therapeutic strategy that is diametrically opposed to the above may be relevant; that is, suppression of both wild-type and mutant alleles without gene augmentation may be appropriate. For certain genes and encoded proteins, significantly reduced levels or indeed complete ablation of endogenous protein may be well tolerated allowing the retina to function normally. In such scenarios, suppression alone of both wild-type and mutant alleles may provide benefit by reducing levels of mutant protein (in parallel with reducing wild-type protein) thereby moderating the toxicity induced by the mutant.

4.3 Gene Suppression Methodologies

Gene suppression and gene augmentation whether required individually (either suppression or replacement) or as a dual-component therapy (suppression and replacement), depending on the mechanism underlying the dominant mutation, in principle, provide rational strategies to treat dominant conditions targeting the primary defect.

If the therapy requires gene suppression, either alone or indeed in combination with gene supplementation, molecular tools to orchestrate potent suppression are essential. A significant challenge has been the absence of methods for suppression of gene expression whose potency was retained from in vitro testing to in vivo studies. While early suppression technologies employed antisense and ribozyme-based molecules, typically, in vivo potency remained an issue (Miyagishi et al. 2003). The advent of RNA interference (RNAi) technologies, with in vivo potency demonstrated in diverse species from *C. elegans* to mammals including primates, provided a novel and powerful molecular tool to orchestrate gene suppression (Fire et al. 1998). RNAi utilizes double-stranded RNA (dsRNA) molecules to suppress gene expression in a sequence-specific manner. It exploits an endogenous cellular machinery involved in processing a wide range of endogenously expressed noncoding RNAs using an armament of components including the RNA-induced silencing complex (RISC) among others (Fagard et al. 2000; Zamore et al. 2000; Bernstein et al. 2001; Hannon 2002; Lee et al. 2004; Tijsterman and Plasterk 2004). Noncoding RNAs processed by the RNAi machinery are central to controlling gene expression and influence developmental programs, cellular homeostasis, and maintenance of chromatin structures, among other activities, and hence, RNAi represents not solely a potent suppressor that can be provided exogenously to modulate gene expression but an endogenous mechanism central to cellular functioning and integrity. With regard to potency and longevity, synthesized RNAi can be chemically modified to increase longevity and to optimize cell transfection or viral and nonviral vectors can provide a sustained supply of RNAi-based suppression (Burnett and Rossi 2012; Bhavsar et al. 2012; Bramsen and Kjems 2013). In parallel, methodologies to minimize risk of toxicity associated with off-target effects of RNAi and/or recruitment and saturation of the endogenous cellular machinery have been developed (Birmingham et al. 2007; Jackson and Linsley 2010; Boudreau et al. 2013). Recently, single-stranded RNAi (ssRNAi) has been used to recruit the endogenous RNAi machinery and in principle

should eliminate the risk of the sense strand of dsRNA entering RISC thereby minimizing potential off-targets (Lima et al. 2012; Liu et al. 2013).

The goal of targeted gene suppression has been achieved with a variety of additional novel technologies. Suppression can be targeted toward transcripts as per the RNAi technologies described above. Alternatively, suppression can be directed toward DNA sequences or encoded proteins. Such approaches can involve modulation of transcription or technologies to elicit correction of DNA or RNA. Molecules available to achieve this include zinc finger proteins (ZFPs), oligonucleotides to induce DNA correction, aptamers, antibodies, transcription activator-like effector nucleases (TALENs), and clustered regulatory interspaced short palindromic repeat (CRISPR)/Cas-based RNA-guided DNA endonucleases among others (Gaj et al. 2013). For example, DNA-binding ZFPs can be used (alone or in conjunction with endonucleases for DNA cleavage) to bind specific DNA targets. Designer peptides incorporating DNA-binding domains consisting of tandem zinc fingers to facilitate binding to specific DNA sequences can be characterized from libraries of ZFPs. The effect(s) of ZFP binding can in turn be controlled such that ZFPs can be used to suppress or induce gene expression by conjugation of ZFPs to repressor or enhancer molecules. Many ZFPs have been designed to bind to 5' promoter sequences of a gene and thereby suppress expression of the target gene. Similarly, targeted correction of a range of genetic mutations has been achieved in cell culture using various nucleases including zinc finger nucleases and TALEN nucleases to introduce double-strand breaks at specific locations and to thereby induce homologous recombination and DNA correction at those locations using exogenously provided DNA fragments (Greenwald et al. 2010; Overlack et al. 2012; Low et al. 2014).

A variety of the suppression technologies outlined above such as antisense, ribozymes, RNAi, and ZFPs has been employed to achieve suppression of genes causative of dominantly inherited retinal degenerations – examples are provided in the chapter (Table 4.1). In principle, the armament of suppressors detailed above could be

Table 4.1 Examples of gene therapies in the development for autosomal dominantly inherited retinal degenerations targeting the primary genetic defect

Preclinical studies

Disease	Gene	Therapeutic approach	Vector	Animal model	Efficacy assessment	References
Autosomal dominant						
Best disease, autosomal dominant	*Best1*	Gene replacement	AAV2	*cmr* dogs, wild-type dogs	ERG, histology	Guziewicz et al. (2013)
Retinitis pigmentosa, autosomal dominant (adRP)	*Prph2 (Rds/peripherin)*	Gene replacement, also suppression and replacement	Compacted DNA nanoparticles, AAV1, AAV2, AAV5	*Prph2(Rd2/Rd2)* null mouse	ERG, histology, cell culture, PCR	Schlichtenbrede et al. (2003), Georgiadis et al. (2010), Cai et al. (2010), Petrs-Silva et al. (2012)
Retinitis pigmentosa, autosomal dominant (adRP)	*RHO*	Suppression and replacement, suppression, zinc finger transcription factors, gene replacement	AAV2	*RHO* P23H rat, *RHO* P347S transgenic mouse, *RHO* P23H mouse	ERG, histology, cell culture	LaVail et al. (2000), Lewin et al. (1998), Gorbatyuk et al. (2005, 2007), O'Reilly et al. (2007). Chadderton et al. (2009), Palfi et al. (2010), Millington-Ward et al. (2011), Mussolino et al. (2011), Mao et al. (2011, 2012), Greenwald et al. (2013)
Cone-rod dystrophy, autosomal dominant (CORD)	*GCAP1*	Suppression of mutant and wild-type genes	Self-complementary AAV8	*GCAP1* L151F transgenic mouse	ERG, histology, cell culture	Jiang et al. (2013)

deployed to moderate the expression of genes directly causative of dominant ocular conditions or to suppress the expression of genes implicated in driving features of the disease which exacerbate the disease pathology.

4.4 Targeting Primary Genetic Defects

Knowledge of the primary genetic mutations underlying dominantly inherited ocular conditions, the availability of potent methods to suppress gene expression, methods of gene delivery such as recombinant adeno-associated viral (AAV) vectors, and, for some retinopathies, the generation of transgenic animals simulating the disorder have provided a platform to explore gene therapies targeted toward correcting the primary genetic lesions. Rhodopsin-linked autosomal dominant RP (*RHO*-adRP) accounts for about 25–30 % of cases of autosomal dominant RP (adRP) and hence is one of the most prevalent forms of RP (Sung et al. 1991; Dryja et al. 1991; Inglehearn et al. 1992). Significant mutational heterogeneity has been characterized in human *RHO*-adRP with approximately 200 disease-causing mutations identified thus far in the RHO gene (Fig. 4.2). Rhodopsin is a highly expressed G protein-coupled receptor in rod photoreceptors and decorates the rod outer segment disc membranes, comprising approximately 90 % of the proteins found in

these membranes (Corless et al. 1982; Hargrave 2001). Transgenically generated rhodopsin null mice (Rho−/−) (Humphries et al. 1997; Lem et al. 1999) present with abnormal retinal function and do not elaborate rod outer segments, thus highlighting the essential role of rhodopsin in the mammalian retina. Given the extensive mutational diversity characteristic of *RHO*-adRP, therapies directed to specific mutant alleles would not be practical involving preclinical and clinical evaluation of many different suppressors, each targeting a specific *RHO* mutation. Furthermore, the observation that Rho−/− mice have a severe pathology suggests that suppression alone, if sufficient suppression were achieved, would be detrimental. Together these data suggest that exploration of suppression of *RHO* in conjunction with gene supplementation, using a replacement gene refractory to suppression, might be a viable therapeutic strategy for this dominantly inherited retinopathy. This strategy would enable a single therapy to correct the defect independent of the precise RHO mutation. Employing features of the genome such as codon redundancy enables the generation of replacement genes (encoding wild-type protein) whose transcripts are refractory to suppression and provide a means of condensing the vast mutational heterogeneity in dominant disorders such as *RHO*-adRP such that a single therapeutic corrects the primary dominant genetic defect albeit requiring a dual-component therapy, suppression and replacement.

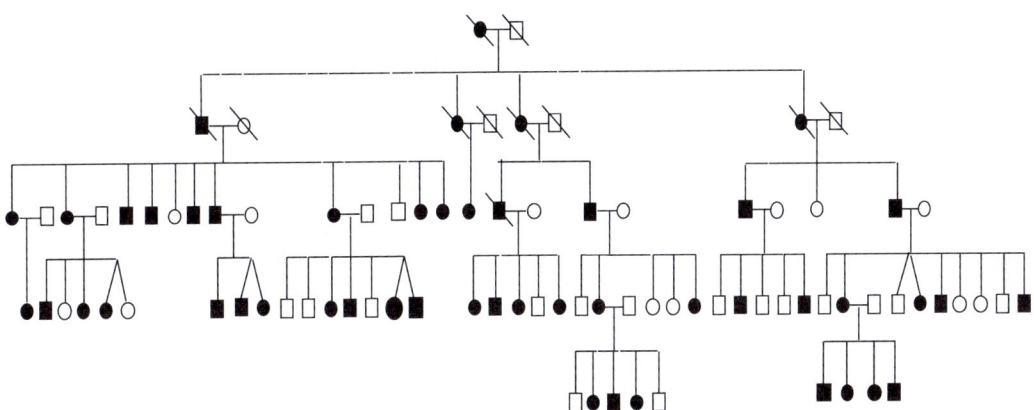

Fig. 4.2 adRP pedigree used to localize RHO-adRP gene. The adRP genes causative of the retinopathies found in patients presented in Fig 4.1 were localized using genetic linkage studies in large adRP pedigrees. For example, the pedigree employed to localize the RHO-adRP gene to 3q is presented here

Transgenic murine models of *RHO*-adRP engineered to express a mutant human *RHO* transgene (Pro347Ser and Pro23His mice) and *Rho−/−* mice were used to explore the approach. The development of a gene-based medicine with two components is challenging; nevertheless, it is likely that therapies with dual modalities will be employed in the future. Indeed already, the combination of gene replacement with the provision of neurotrophic factors has been explored for some forms of retinal degeneration (Buch et al. 2006; Komáromy et al. 2013). Hence, to dissect the efficacy of each of the individual components of this dual-acting therapeutic to correct *RHO*-adRP mutations involving RNAi-mediated suppression and gene replacement, RNAi suppressors were generated which target human *RHO* but leave mouse *Rho* intact by exploiting the sequence divergence of the rhodopsin DNA sequence between the two species. Indeed, a similar strategy has been adopted in assessing RNAi-based therapies for other neurodegenerative conditions, such as spinocerebellar ataxia (SCA) and Huntington's disease (HD), where the endogenous mouse genes have acted as replacement genes refractory to suppression due to nucleotide sequence divergence between species (Xia et al. 2004; Harper et al. 2005).

As briefly described above, the vector of choice for these studies was AAV, and in particular AAV serotype 5 was employed; however, alternative AAV serotypes such as AAV7 and AAV8 which also transduce photoreceptors efficiently (Vandenberghe et al. 2013) could be utilized. 2×10^9 vg of AAV2/5 vectors, which expressed RNAi targeting human RHO, was subretinally injected into RHO P347S mice, and effects of suppression of human mutant *RHO* were observed. Indeed, significant benefit was derived from single subretinal injections as evaluated by retinal histology and electroretinography, however, noting, as stated above, that in this case the endogenous rhodopsin gene acts as a replacement gene (Chadderton et al. 2009).

In parallel with the suppression studies, which demonstrated proof of concept of the RNAi-based element of the therapy, it was imperative to generate a *RHO* replacement vector, which was refractory to RNAi-mediated suppression. The replacement vector would have to supply sufficient doses of wild-type RHO protein to compensate for the suppression of both the wild-type and mutant alleles of human *RHO* that would occur in the final therapeutic combining suppression and replacement. The *RHO* gene, as eluded to above, is highly expressed in rod photoreceptors (Corless et al. 1982), hence, recapitulating high levels of *RHO* expression from a viral vector required evaluation of a family of vectors (Palfi et al. 2010). The Rho−/− null mouse was used to explore the potency of *RHO* gene replacement constructs. Significant engineering of the *RHO* promoter resulted in the production of AAV2/5 vectors incorporating a rhodopsin promoter-driven *RHO* replacement gene, the latter modified over the target site for suppression employing the degeneracy of the genetic code. A single subretinal injection of 6×10^9 vg of virus resulted in significant rescue of the phenotype characteristic of the Rho−/− null mouse (Palfi et al. 2010).

Given the demonstration of proof of concept of each of the individual components of RNAi suppression and codon-modified gene replacement, the dual components were combined and *RHO*-adRP suppression and replacement therapies explored in P347S mice. In this case, an RNAi suppressor that targeted both mouse and human rhodopsin was used to simulate the situation that would occur in human patients where both mutant and wild-type alleles would be suppressed. After a single subretinal injection of two AAV vectors, one expressing the suppressor and the other the codon-modified and optimized replacement gene, significant benefit was observed using histological and electrophysiological readouts (Millington-Ward et al. 2011). The approach represents a gene therapy which targets the primary dominant defect in a mutation-independent manner thereby overcoming the significant mutational diversity characteristic of many dominantly inherited disorders and hence is not limited to application in ocular conditions but is relevant to many diseases. With regard to ocular disorders, the strategy of suppression and replacement is being assessed for dominant retinopathies including *RHO*-adRP as detailed above and peripherin-linked adRP (Palfi et al. 2006; Georgiadis et al. 2010). Genable Technologies is focused on progressing suppression and replacement based gene therapies to the clinic to provide novel and effective therapeutic solutions for dominantly inherited disorders. As the approach holds broad applicability for many dominant conditions involving mutational heterogeneity and requiring, or benefiting from, continued expression (or where appropriate overexpression) of the wild-type protein, it is likely that the technology will be used to design therapies for many disorders in the next few years. Indeed, neurodegenerative disorders such as spinocerebellar ataxia (SCA) or Huntington's disease (HD) among others may be suited to such a therapeutic strategy (Keiser et al. 2013). While promising, the strategy involves dual components and hence will require considerable optimization to ensure potent suppression of the target gene in conjunction with sufficient expression of the replacement gene, as outlined in the experiments detailed above.

An alternative approach to treating dominant disorders that may be relevant where haploinsufficiency accounts for at least some of the disease pathology is delivery of the wild-type gene alone (Table 4.1). Indeed, in this regard, Mao et al. (2011) delivered the wild-type *RHO* gene to mice and obtained histological and ERG benefit in a P23H knock-in mouse model of *RHO*-adRP (Sakami et al. 2011). More recently, AAV has been employed to deliver the *BEST1* gene encoding bestrophin to a recessive canine model of Best disease, a macular degeneration that can be inherited either recessively or dominantly. It remains to be elucidated if gene augmentation alone will be relevant to both recessive and dominant forms of this condition (Guziewicz et al. 2013).

In contrast to the above, certain wild-type proteins may not be required for normal functioning of retinal neurons. "Suppression only" involving suppression of both wild-type and mutant alleles may provide a viable therapeutic strategy for dominant diseases involving such genes. *IMPDH1*-linked adRP is a relatively severe form of RP, and yet the *Impdh1* knockout mouse has an extremely mild phenotype suggesting that absence or reduced levels of IMPDH1 may be tolerated in the mammalian retina. Therefore, for *IMPDH1*-adRP, a suppression only strategy may provide benefit as demonstrated in an RNAi-induced mouse model of *IMPDH1*-adRP (Tam et al. 2008; Table 4.1). The findings of beneficial effects associated with gene replacement alone and suppression alone therapies have also been mirrored in neurodegenerative diseases of the brain. For example, each of these single therapeutic strategies has been found to provide benefit in mouse models of SCA. Indeed, the recent study by Keiser et al. (2013) demonstrating that suppression and gene augmentation separately are beneficial in SCA stimulates the question as to whether combining both strategies, that is, employing both suppression and replacement together by using replacement genes resistant to suppression as described above for *RHO*-adRP, may augment the benefit. Undoubtedly, the features of the human genome, such as codon redundancy, which enable the development of such therapies for dominant conditions, will be employed over the coming years.

RHO suppression with the ultimate objective of incorporating such suppressors as components of gene therapies for *RHO*-adRP has been achieved using a variety of molecules including RNAi as recorded above, ribozymes (LaVail et al. 2000), and ZNFs (Mussolino et al. 2011). Indeed, a number of studies have employed ribozymes to suppress mutant and wild-type rhodopsin alleles utilizing the sequence discrimination that can be achieved with ribozymes, catalytic RNA enzymes that cleave target transcripts in a sequence-specific manner using antisense arms to guide the RNA enzyme to the target sequence (LaVail et al. 2000). Employing the P347S mouse model of *RHO*-adRP, an AAV vector encoding a ZFP targeting the promoter sequence of the *RHO* gene was found to provide benefit by suppression of the mutant P347S *RHO*; for these proof of concept studies, expression of the endogenous mouse rhodopsin gene was employed to provide wild-type rhodopsin protein (Mussolino et al. 2011; Table 4.1). Undoubtedly, DNA correction technologies will be explored more extensively in the context of correcting inherited retinopathies (both recessive and dominant) over the next few years as the precision, resolution, and efficacy of such methodologies are optimized. Indeed, it is notable that application of TALEN technology is starting to emerge for inherited retinopathies (Low et al. 2014), albeit for a recessive retinopathy, the Crb1 (rd8) mutation. Correction of the Crb1 (rd8) retinopathy in mice generated from fertilized oocytes co-injected with a TALEN-based nuclease targeting the Crb1 (rd8) allele, together with oligonucleotides to correct the mutant allele, occurred in approximately 27 % of offspring; heterozygous mice with one corrected allele had a normal retinal phenotype (Low et al. 2014). Close monitoring and minimization of modification at off-target sites will be essential for such DNA correction technologies.

As stated above it is likely that dual-component therapies, whether involving suppression and replacement, or therapies modulating other features of disease such as neuronal longevity, oxidative stress, or other disease mechanisms (see section below) will be explored extensively in the future. To implement these strategies, the ability to coinfect target cells with more than a single AAV vector will be extremely valuable. In this regard, coinfection of photoreceptors after subretinal delivery of AAV-EGFP and AAV-DsRed reporter vectors has been explored (Fig. 4.3) for both AAV2/5 and AAV2/8 serotypes and considerable levels of cotransduc-

tion achieved in photoreceptors (Palfi et al. 2012; Trapani et al. 2014).

For many dominantly inherited mutations, the precise mode of action remains to be elucidated fully, representing an additional complication in the development of therapies for such disorders. Deciphering the mechanism by which the mutation is causative of the disease should enable the optimal therapeutic strategy to be chosen when considering potential treatments. Furthermore, elucidation of the modes of action of dominant mutations and their downstream effects may provide additional novel pathways for therapeutic development. The modulation of pathways common between different dominantly inherited retinal degenerations may potentially provide beneficial effects as outlined in the section below.

4.5   Targeting Secondary Effects

The characterization of common pathways of disease pathology in retinal dystrophies with diverse genetic etiologies has provided insights to the key components driving disease processes. While of fundamental biological interest in terms of exploring the molecular mechanisms underlying the disorders, the observation of similar features between genetically distinct retinal disorders has also prompted exploration of novel therapeutic strategies with potentially broad applicability. The development of more generic therapies is particularly attractive for inherited

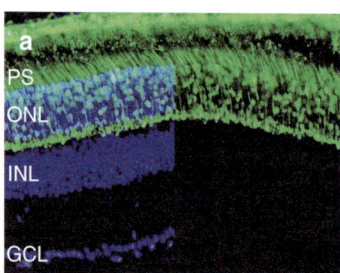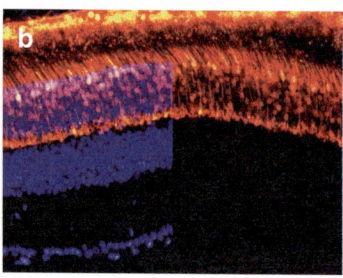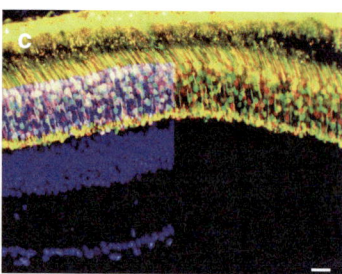

Fig. 4.3 **EGFP and DsRed reporter co-transduction using AAV2/5 in the mouse retina**. Eyes of adult 129 wild-type mice were subretinally injected with a mixture of 1.5 x10⁹ vg of AAV-CMVP-EGFP and 1.5x10⁹ vg of AAV-CMVP-DsRed AAV. Two weeks post-injection, eyes were fixed, cryosectioned and counterstained with DAPI. Composite microscope images illustrate the native fluorescence of reporter proteins. (**a**) EGFP signal, (**b**) DsRed signal, (**c**) EGFP and DsRed signals overlaid. Note that the left half of the images was overlaid with DAPI signal. *GCL* ganglion cell layer, *INL* inner nuclear layer, *ONL* outer nuclear layer, *PS* photoreceptor segment layer. Scale bar: 25 μm (panel C)

Table 4.2 Therapeutic strategies for retinitis pigmentosa (RP) targeting secondary effects associated with the disease pathology

Gene or protein	Therapeutic approach	Vector	Animal model	Efficacy assessment	References
SOD1 SOD2, catalase	Antioxidative stress	Transgenically expressed	Rd1 and Rd10 mice	ERG, histology	Usui et al. (2009, 2011)
RdCVF, RdCVF2	Neurotrophic factor	Injection of protein	Rd1 mouse, *RHO* P23H rat	ERG, histology	LeVéillard et al. (2004), Yang et al. (2009), Jaillard et al. (2012)
GDNF, FGF	Neurotrophic factor	Nonviral electrotransfer, AAV-ShH10, transgenically expressed, AAV2	*RHO* S334ter rat, Rd10 mouse, RCSI rat, Rd2 mouse	ERG, histology	Touchard et al. (2012), Dalkara et al. (2011), Ohnaka et al. (2012), Buch et al. (2006)
CNTF	Neurotrophic factor	Injection of protein, transplantation of CNTF-secreting devices, AAV2, encapsulated cell technology	*RHO* S334ter rat, *Rds* P216L mouse, Rd2 mouse, human clinical trial	ERG, histology	Li et al. (2010), Bok et al. (2002), Buch et al. (2006), Birch et al. (2013)
Bip/Grp78Hsf-1	Modulation of the UPR/chaperone	AAV5	*RHO* P23H rat	ERG, histology	Gorbatyuk et al. (2010)
Ablation of Caspase 7	Modulation of the UPR/anti-apoptotic agent	Transgenically assessed	*RHO* T17M mouse, *Casp-7-/-* mouse	ERG, OCT, histology, cell culture	Choudhury et al. (2013)
XIAP	Anti-apoptotic agent	AAV5	*RHO* P23H and S334ter rats	ERG, histology, Western blot	Leonard et al. (2007), Yao et al. (2012)

Examples of gene therapies for autosomal dominant RP (adRP) are provided, together with a number of examples of approaches in the development for autosomal recessive RP (arRP)

retinopathies, given the immense genetic diversity in disease etiology present in these disorders, which has greatly impeded therapeutic development to date. An alternative therapeutic strategy to correcting the primary genetic defect is modulation of the secondary effects associated with the disease course resulting in restoration or preservation of cellular function(s) toward a wild-type phenotype (Trifunović et al. 2012; Athanasiou et al. 2013; Table 4.2). A convergence of potential therapeutic solutions for such etiologically diverse disorders by targeting common features in principle should provide a more readily translatable therapeutic opportunity.

Indeed, similarities in disease mechanisms are characteristic not only of retinal degenerations but, moreover, degenerative disorders of the brain, and hence, it is not surprising that the therapeutic strategies being considered for retinopathies mirror those being explored for other neurodegenerative conditions (Douglas 2013; van den Heuvel et al. 2014). The convergence of disease mechanisms between retinal and brain degenerations provides an opportunity to design innovative treatments that may be relevant to both these broad categories of disease. Tissue-specific transcriptomics from healthy and diseased tissues has demonstrated that some components influencing cell longevity and homeostasis are common to multiple tissues while others show more specific patterns of expression. These observations have stimulated the exploration of broad categories of therapeutics, each of which has evolved into a large field of research and translation medicine. Examples of such strategies are provided below (Tables 4.1 and 4.2). Various neurodegenerative diseases, including dominant retinopathies, have been modulated in preclinical animal models, by overexpression of neurotrophic factors thereby extending neuronal longevity (Touchard et al. 2012; Keifer et al. 2014; Kordower and Bjorklund 2013; Hickey and Stacy 2013). Likewise, therapeutic benefit has been associated with attenuation of oxidative stress causative of cellular damage and compromised survival, provision of anti-apoptotic molecules to modulate programmed cell death, and perturbation of cellular stress responses to aggregated proteins, all of which are damaging insults for neurons. Examples of gene therapies for dominantly inherited retinopathies are detailed in this chapter providing an overview of these emerging fields (Tables 4.1 and 4.2).

4.6   Neurotrophic Factors

Exploration of the therapeutic potential of gene therapies encoding neurotrophic factors for dominant retinopathies was initiated almost two decades ago. Benefit associated with the delivery of neurotrophic factor proteins in the *RHO* Q344ter murine model of *RHO*-adRP and the Rdy cat, a feline model of *CRX*-linked adRP, was reported as early as 1998 and 1999, respectively (LaVail et al. 1998; Chong et al. 1999). Therapeutic benefit in rodent models of RP, as evaluated by histology, electrophysiology, and/or functional assays, has been obtained using neurotrophic factors including rod-derived cone viability factor (RdCVF) in the *RHO* P23H rat (Yang et al. 2009), ciliary neurotrophic factor (CNTF) in a S334ter-3 *RHO*-adRP transgenic rat (Li et al. 2010) and the P216L rds/peripherin mouse (Bok et al. 2002), and glial-derived neurotrophic factor (GDNF) in S334ter rats (Dalkara et al. 2011) and members of the family of fibroblast growth factors (FGF) among many others (Ohnaka et al. 2012; Touchard et al. 2012; Léveillard and Sahel 2010). For example, transgenic (Ohnaka et al. 2012), viral (Buch et al. 2006; Dalkara et al. 2011), and nonviral (Touchard et al. 2012) delivery of GDNF has been shown to be neuroprotective for different cell types within the degenerating mammalian retina. Typically, the studies with neurotrophic factors are at a preclinical stage. However, a therapy utilizing encapsulated cell

technology (ECT; Buch et al. 2004) involving an intravitreal device with cells engineered to overexpress CNTF has progressed to clinical trial for the treatment of RP and AMD (Birch et al. 2013) and included some patients with dominant forms of RP. Results thus far indicated that the device was well tolerated although no beneficial effects for primary outcome measures including visual acuity and visual field sensitivity were obtained. Significant increases in retinal thickness were observed in treated eyes (Birch et al. 2013). For any particular neurotrophic factor, the route of administration, the ability to confine the therapy to the target cell type, together with tight control on dose given the possible pleiotropic effects of the therapies will influence the efficacy of such therapies in human patients.

4.7   Modulating Cellular Stress

Disease mechanisms in common between Mendelian forms of retinopathies and more prevalent retinal degenerations such as AMD include cellular stresses such as oxidative stress, mitochondrial dysfunction, endoplasmic reticulum (ER) stress, and induction of the unfolded protein response and stimulation of apoptotic programs. Each of these processes, either individually or in concert, can stimulate cascades of events, leading to cellular damage and sometimes cell death. One therapeutic strategy for retinopathies is modulation of the levels of oxidative stress in the degenerating retina. As rod photoreceptor cells die in a retina undergoing a progressive rod-cone dystrophy, the remaining cone photoreceptor cells may be subjected to increasing levels of oxygen, promoting oxidative damage to cones. In this regard, cocktails of exogenously delivered antioxidants have been injected into rodent models of RP and beneficial effects on photoreceptor cell density and function observed in treated versus control eyes (Komeima et al. 2007). Alternatively, a transgenic approach has been used to achieve overexpression of superoxide dismutase 2 (*SOD2*) and catalase resulting in reduction in oxidative damage and preservation of cone density in mouse model of RP (Usui et al. 2009, 2011). It is likely that overlapping mechanisms may be involved between neurotrophic and antioxidant therapeutic strategies. For example, RdCVF is a thioredoxin-like protein encoded by the *Nxn1* gene that mediates resistance to photooxidative damage and can protect cone photoreceptors in the rd1 mouse model of recessive RP (Levéillard et al. 2004) and dominant P23H *RHO*-adRP transgenic rat (Yang et al. 2009) as detailed in the section above. The paralogous *Nxn2* gene product RdCVF2 similarly has been found to be protective to cones (Jaillard et al. 2012). The *Nxn1* and *Nxn2* genes both encode short (RdCVF and RdCVF2) and long isoforms (RdCVFL and RdCVFL2) providing elegant examples of how protein diversity can arise through optimal utilization of overlapping coding sequences (Fridlich et al. 2009; Jaillard et al. 2012).

While the provision of neurotrophic factors and modulation of oxidative stress represent therapeutic strategies that potentially could be relevant to many forms of inherited retinopathies, modulation of the cellular events driven by the presence of aggregated proteins represents an additional therapeutic approach that is being explored for some retinal disorders. Indeed, various mutations causative of inherited retinopathies lead to protein misfolding and aggregation, can induce ER stress and the unfolded protein response (UPR), and result in cellular toxicity and potentially apoptosis. With respect to adRP, it is clear that some *RHO* mutations operate in this manner (Griciuc et al. 2011). More generally, aggregated proteins have been implicated in a wide range of neurodegenerations, including Alzheimer's disease, Parkinson's disease, and Huntington's disease among others. Therapies that facilitate chaperoning of misfolded proteins and thereby modulation of ER stress and the UPR are being evaluated in preclinical studies. One approach involves augmentation with protein chaperones. Indeed, with respect to dominant retinopathies, AAV-delivered overexpression of a gene encoding a chaperone termed *Grp78/BiP* provided preservation of photoreceptor function in P23H *RHO*-adRP rats (Gorbatyuk et al. 2010). Small molecules have also been explored, for

example, 17-AAG, an inhibitor of heat shock protein (HSP) 90 and an inducer of HSP70, was found to be protective in an AAV-induced mouse model of *IMPDH1*-adRP (Tam et al. 2010). In a recent study, small molecule inhibitors, HSP990 and 17-AAG, targeting HSP90, have been evaluated in two rat models of *RHO*-adRP, the P23H and P135L models. While the strategy provided benefit in these *RHO*-adRP models, it was noted that sustained expression may potentially modulate proteins involved in retinal function, for example, sustained treatment with HSP990, resulted in reductions in GRK1 and PDE6 (Aguilà et al. 2014). In an attempt to modulate the UPR and downstream effects such as apoptosis, Gorbatyuk and colleagues explored the therapeutic potential of ablation of caspase 7 in a mouse model of *RHO*-adRP, the T17M mouse, and observed the substantial preservation of photoreceptor cells and visual function as a result of caspase 7 ablation (Choudhury et al. 2013).

Apoptosis may be considered as the final stage in the life cycle of retinal cells in a degenerating retina irrespective of the primary insult driving the degenerative process such as light excitotoxicity, oxidative stress, presence of aggregated proteins, etc. (Doonan et al. 2012). As per the processes detailed above, apoptosis represents a common pathway that may be modulated to develop therapeutics with potentially broad applicability. Light-induced retinal degeneration in rodents has provided key insights into the molecular mechanisms underlying apoptosis (Hao et al. 2002). While caspases frequently play central roles in apoptosis (Perche et al. 2007), caspase-independent mechanisms can also be involved during photoreceptor apoptosis (Sano et al. 2006; Doonan et al. 2003). Elevation of intracellular calcium ions and participation of calpains play an important role in some forms of retinal apoptosis (Marigo 2007; Nakazawa 2011). Knowledge regarding key components driving apoptotic pathways in the degenerating retina has provided targets for anti-apoptotic gene therapies. For example, the X-linked inhibitor of apoptosis (*XIAP*, a caspase inhibitor) has undergone preclinical testing in *RHO*-adRP rodent models; AAV-*XIAP* has been found to be protective for photoreceptors in *RHO* P23H and S334ter RP rats (Leonard et al. 2002). The same approach (AAV-XIAP) has been explored as an adjunct to an AAV-mediated gene replacement therapy and found to augment the efficacy of the replacement therapy (Yao et al. 2012).

It is notable that for many neurodegenerative disorders, including retinopathies, involvement at some level of mitochondrial dysfunction has been established (Farrar et al. 2013) and indeed interplays with many of the processes detailed above such as oxidative stress. Therapies targeted at modulating mitochondrial function are being explored, and undoubtedly, this type of approach will be investigated in greater detail over the next few years. Is it clear that a wide variety of different but potentially synergistic therapeutic approaches are being considered for inherited retinal degenerations, including dominantly inherited forms of these conditions as detailed above (Table 4.2). Therapies may be directed toward correcting the primary dominant genetic defect underlying the disease process or may be targeted at modulating secondary effects associated with these retinopathies. Therapies may be provided alone, or potentially as combination therapies, as detailed above. It would seem likely that as the field matures, multivalent therapies addressing multiple features characteristic of these disorders may be employed to optimize beneficial effects.

Conclusions

Therapeutic strategies that are being considered for retinal degenerations, with a particular focus on dominant forms of these conditions, have been outlined in this chapter. Therapeutic avenues being explored for dominant retinopathies include targeting the primary genetic defect or modulation of secondary effects associated with the disease pathology. Approaches in the development to correct the primary genetic defect underlying retinal degenerations such as *RHO*-adRP have been detailed in this chapter. It may be that combination therapies involving more than one approach will ultimately provide optimal

benefit. A therapy directed toward correcting the primary defect in conjunction with additional active component(s) such as provision of a neurotrophic factor may augment potency of therapies. In this regard, there is significant interplay between the various therapeutic strategies being addressed. For example, the provision of neurotrophic factors can operate via multiple mechanisms and can potentially modulate apoptosis, oxidative stress, mitochondrial function, and/or deleterious effects due to protein aggregation. The coming decade undoubtedly will witness many of the therapies in the categories outlined above, which are currently in preclinical studies, progressing into the clinic.

Compliance with Ethical Requirements
Conflict of Interest G Jane Farrar is a Director and Paul F. Kenna is an Observer of Genable Technologies Ltd. Sophia Millington-Ward, Arpad Palfi, and Naomi Chadderton are consultants of Genable Technologies Ltd.

Informed Consent No human studies were carried out by the authors for this article.

Animal Studies No animal studies were carried out by the authors for this article.

References

Aguilà M, Bevilacqua D, McCulley C et al (2014) Hum Mol Genet 23(8):2164–2175
Athanasiou D, Aguilà M, Bevilacqua D et al (2013) The cell stress machinery and retinal degeneration. FEBS Lett 587(13):2008–2017
Audo I, Bujakowska KM, Léveillard T et al (2012) Development and application of a next-generation-sequencing (NGS) approach to detect known and novel gene defects underlying retinal diseases. Orphanet J Rare Dis 7:8
Ayuso C, Millan JM (2010) Retinitis pigmentosa and allied conditions today: a paradigm of translational research. Genome Med 2:34
Bainbridge JW, Smith AJ, Barker SS et al (2008) Effect of gene therapy on visual function in Leber's congenital amaurosis. N Engl J Med 358:2231–2239
Bernstein E, Caudy AA, Hammond SM, Hannon GJ et al (2001) Role for a bidentate ribonuclease in the initiation step of RNA interference. Nature 409:363–366
Bhattacharya SS, Wright AF, Clayton JF et al (1984) Close genetic linkage between X-linked retinitis

pigmentosa and a restriction fragment length polymorphism identified by recombinant DNA probe L1.28. Nature 309:253–255

Bhavsar D, Subramanian K, Sethuraman S et al (2012) Translational siRNA therapeutics using liposomal carriers: prospects & challenges. Curr Gene Ther 4:315–332

Birch DG, Weleber RG, Duncan JL et al (2013) Randomized trial of ciliary neurotrophic factor delivered by encapsulated cell intraocular implants for retinitis pigmentosa. Am J Ophthalmol 156(2):283–292

Birmingham A, Anderson E, Sullivan K et al (2007) A protocol for designing siRNAs with high functionality and specificity. Nat Protoc 2:2068–2078

Bok D, Yasumura D, Matthes MT et al (2002) Effects of adeno-associated virus-vectored ciliary neurotrophic factor on retinal structure and function in mice with a P216L rds/peripherin mutation. Exp Eye Res 74: 719–735

Boudreau RL, Spengler RM, Hylock RH et al (2013) siSPOTR: a tool for designing highly specific and potent siRNAs for human and mouse. Nucleic Acids Res 41(1):e9

Bowne SJ, Sullivan LS, Koboldt DC et al (2011) Identification of disease-causing mutations in autosomal dominant retinitis pigmentosa (adRP) using next-generation DNA sequencing. Invest Ophthalmol Vis Sci 52:494–504

Bramsen JB, Kjems J (2013) Engineering small interfering RNAs by strategic chemical modification. Methods Mol Biol 942:87–109

Buch RA, Lei B, Tao W et al (2004) Encapsulated cell-based intraocular delivery of ciliary neurotrophic factor in normal rabbit: dose-dependent effects on ERG and retinal histology. Invest Ophthalmol Vis Sci 45:2420–2430

Buch PK, MacLaren RE, Durán Y et al (2006) In contrast to AAV-mediated Cntf expression, AAV-mediated Gdnf expression enhances gene replacement therapy in rodent models of retinal degeneration. Mol Ther 14:700–709

Burnett JC, Rossi JJ (2012) RNA-based therapeutics: current progress and future prospects. Chem Biol 19(1):60–71

Cai X, Conley SM, Naash MI (2010) Gene therapy in the Retinal Degeneration Slow model of retinitis pigmentosa. Adv Exp Med Biol 664:611–619

Chadderton N, Millington-Ward S, Palfi A et al (2009) Improved retinal function in a mouse model of dominant retinitis pigmentosa following AAV-delivered gene therapy. Mol Ther 17:593–599

Choi M, Scholl UI, Ji W et al (2009) Genetic diagnosis by whole exome capture and massively parallel DNA sequencing. Proc Natl Acad Sci U S A 106:19096–19101

Chong NH, Alexander RA, Waters L et al (1999) Repeated injections of a ciliary neurotrophic factor analogue leading to long-term photoreceptor survival in hereditary retinal degeneration. Invest Ophthalmol Vis Sci 40:1298–1305

Choudhury S, Bhootada Y, Gorbatyuk O, Gorbatyuk M (2013) Caspase-7 ablation modulates UPR, reprograms TRAF2-JNK apoptosis and protects T17M rhodopsin mice from severe retinal degeneration. Cell Death Dis 4:e528

Cideciyan AV, Aleman TS, Boye SL et al (2008) Human gene therapy for RPE65 isomerase deficiency activates the retinoid cycle of vision but with slow rod kinetics. Proc Natl Acad Sci U S A 105: 15112–15117

Corless JM, McCaslin DR, Scott B (1982) Two-dimensional rhodopsin crystals from disk membranes of frog retinal rod outer segments. Proc Natl Acad Sci U S A 79:1116–1120

Craig DW, Pearson JV, Szelinger S et al (2008) Identification of genetic variants using bar-coded multiplexed sequencing. Nat Methods 5(10):887–893

Dalkara D, Kolstad KD, Guerin KI et al (2011) AAV mediated GDNF secretion from retinal glia slows down retinal degeneration in a rat model of retinitis pigmentosa. Mol Ther 19(9):1602–1608

Doonan F, Donovan M, Cotter TG (2003) Caspase-independent photoreceptor apoptosis in mouse models of retinal degeneration. J Neurosci 23(13): 5723–5731

Doonan F, Groeger G, Cotter TG (2012) Preventing retinal apoptosis–is there a common therapeutic theme? Exp Cell Res 318(11):1278–1284

Douglas MR (2013) Gene therapy for Parkinson's disease: state-of-the-art treatments for neurodegenerative disease. Expert Rev Neurother 13(6):695–705

Dryja TP, McGee TL, Reichel E et al (1990) A point mutation of the rhodopsin gene in one form of retinitis pigmentosa. Nature 343:364–366

Dryja TP, Hahn LB, Cowley GS et al (1991) Mutation spectrum of the rhodopsin gene omong patients with autosomal dominant retinitis pigmentosa. Proc Natl Acad Sci U S A 88:9370–9374

Fagard M, Boutet S, Morel JB et al (2000) AGO1, QDE-2, and RDE-1 are related proteins required for post-transcriptional gene silencing in plants, quelling in fungi, and RNA interference in animals. Proc Natl Acad Sci U S A 2000(97):11650–11654

Farrar GJ, McWilliam P, Bradley DG et al (1990) Autosomal dominant retinitis pigmentosa: linkage to rhodopsin and evidence for genetic heterogeneity. Genomics 8:35–40

Farrar GJ, Kenna P, Jordan SA et al (1991) A three-base-pair deletion in the peripherin-RDS gene in one form of retinitis pigmentosa. Nature 354:478–480

Farrar GJ, Chadderton N, Kenna PF, Millington-Ward S (2013) Mitochondrial disorders: aetiologies, models systems, and candidate therapies. Trends Genet 29(8):488–497

Farrar GJ, Millington-Ward S, Chadderton N, Mansergh FC, Palfi A (2014) Gene therapies for inherited retinal disorders. Vis Neurosci 31(4–5):289–307

Fauser S, Munz M, Besch D (2003) Further support for digenic inheritance in Bardet-Biedl syndrome. J Med Genet 40:e104

Ferrari S, Di Iorio E, Barbaro V, Ponzin D, Sorrentino FS, Parmeggiani F (2011) Retinitis pigmentosa: genes and disease mechanisms. Curr Genomics 12(4):238–249

Fire A, Xu S, Montgomery MK et al (1998) Potent and specific genetic interference by double-stranded RNA in Caenorhabditis elegans. Nature 391:806–811

Fridlich R, Delalande F, Jaillard C et al (2009) The thioredoxin-like protein rod-derived cone viability factor (RdCVFL) interacts with TAU and inhibits its phosphorylation in the retina. Mol Cell Proteomics 8:1206–1218

Gaj T, Gersbach CA, Barbas CF (2013) ZFN, TALEN, and CRISPR/Cas-based methods for genome engineering. Trends Biotechnol 31:397–405

Georgiadis A, Tschernutter M, Bainbridge JWB et al (2010) AAV-mediated knockdown of peripherin-2 in vivo using miRNA-based hairpins. Gene Ther 17:486–493

Glöckle N, Kohl S, Mohr J et al (2014) Panel-based next generation sequencing as a reliable and efficient technique to detect mutations in unselected patients with retinal dystrophies. Eur J Hum Genet 22:99–104

Gorbatyuk MS, Pang JJ, Thomas J Jr et al (2005) Knockdown of wild-type mouse rhodopsin using an AAV vectored ribozyme as part of an RNA replacement approach. Mol Vis 11:648–656

Gorbatyuk M, Justilien V, Liu J et al (2007) Preservation of photoreceptor morphology and function in P23H rats using an allele independent ribozyme. Exp Eye Res 84:44–52

Gorbatyuk MS, Knox T, LaVail MM et al (2010) Restoration of visual function in P23H rhodopsin transgenic rats by gene delivery of BiP/Grp78. Proc Natl Acad Sci U S A 107:5961–5966

Greenwald DL, Cashman SM, Kumar-Singh R (2010) Engineered zinc finger nuclease-mediated homologous recombination of the human rhodopsin gene. Invest Ophthalmol Vis Sci 51:6374–6380

Greenwald DL, Cashman SM, Kumar-Singh R (2013) Mutation-independent rescue of a novel mouse model of Retinitis Pigmentosa. Gene Ther 20(4):425–434

Griciuc A, Aron L, Ueffing M (2011) ER stress in retinal degeneration: a target for rational therapy? Trends Mol Med 17(8):442–451

Guziewicz KE, Zangerl B, Komáromy AM, Iwabe S, Chiodo VA, Boye SL, Hauswirth WW, Beltran WA, Aguirre GD (2013) Recombinant AAV-mediated BEST1 transfer to the retinal pigment epithelium: analysis of serotype-dependent retinal effects. PLoS One 8(10):e75666

Hannon GJ (2002) RNA interference. Nature 418:244–251

Hao W, Wenzel A, Obin MS et al (2002) Evidence for two apoptotic pathways in light-induced retinal degeneration. Nat Genet 32(2):254–260

Hargrave PA (2001) Rhodopsin structure, function, and topography the Friedenwald lecture. Invest Ophthalmol Vis Sci 42:3–9

Harper SQ, Staber PD, He X et al (2005) RNA interference improves motor and neuropathological abnormalities in a Huntington's disease mouse model. Proc Natl Acad Sci U S A 102:5820–5825

Hickey P, Stacy M (2013) AAV2-neurturin (CERE-120) for Parkinson's disease. Expert Opin Biol Ther 13:137–145

Howell N, Bindoff LA, McCullough DA et al (1991) Leber hereditary optic neuropathy: identification of the same mitochondrial ND1 mutation in six pedigrees. Am J Hum Genet 49:939–950

Humphries MM, Rancourt D, Farrar GJ et al (1997) Retinopathy induced in mice by targeted disruption of the rhodopsin gene. Nat Genet 15:216–219

Inglehearn CF, Keen TJ, Bashir R et al (1992) A completed screen for mutations of the rhodopsin gene in a panel of patients with autosomal dominant retinitis pigmentosa. Hum Mol Genet 1:41–45

Jackson AL, Linsley PS (2010) Recognizing and avoiding siRNA off-target effects for target identification and therapeutic application. Nat Rev Drug Discov 9:57–67

Jaillard C, Mouret A, Niepon ML et al (2012) Nxnl2 splicing results in dual functions in neuronal cell survival and maintenance of cell integrity. Hum Mol Genet 21(10):2298–2311

Jiang L, Li TZ, Boye SE, Hauswirth WW et al (2013) RNAi-mediated gene suppression in a GCAP1(L151F) cone-rod dystrophy mouse model. PLoS One 8(3): e57676

Kajiwara K, Hahn LB, Mukai S et al (1991) Mutation in the human retinal degeneration slow gene in autosomal dominant retinitis pigmentosa. Nature 354:480–483

Kajiwara K, Berson EL, Dryja TP (1994) Digenic retinitis pigmentosa due to mutations at the unlinked peripherin/RDS and ROM1 loci. Science 264:1604–1608

Keifer OP Jr, O'Connor DM, Boulis NM et al (2014) Gene and protein therapies utilizing VEGF for ALS. Pharmacol Ther 141:261–271

Keiser MS, Geoghegan JC, Boudreau RL et al (2013) RNAi or overexpression: alternative therapies for Spinocerebellar Ataxia Type 1. Neurobiol Dis 56:6–13

Komáromy AM, Rowlan JS, Corr AT et al (2013) Transient photoreceptor deconstruction by CNTF enhances rAAV-mediated cone functional rescue in late stage CNGB3-achromatopsia. Mol Ther 21(6):1131–1141

Komeima K, Rogers BS, Campochiaro PA (2007) Antioxidants slow photoreceptor cell death in mouse models of retinitis pigmentosa. J Cell Physiol 213:809–815

Kordower JH, Bjorklund A (2013) Trophic factor gene therapy for Parkinson's disease. Mov Disord 28:96–109

LaVail MM, Yasumura D, Matthes MT et al (1998) Protection of mouse photoreceptors by survival factors in retinal degenerations. Invest Ophthalmol Vis Sci 39:592–602

LaVail MM, Yasumura D, Matthes MT (2000) Ribozyme rescue of photoreceptor cells in P23H transgenic rats:

long-term survival and late-stage therapy. Proc Natl Acad Sci U S A 97:11488–11493

Leanaers G, Hamel C, Delettre C et al (2012) Dominant optic atrophy. Orphanet J Rare Dis 7:46

Lee YS, Nakahara K, Pham JW et al (2004) Distinct roles for Drosophila Dicer-1 and Dicer-2 in the siRNA/miRNA silencing pathways. Cell 117:69–81

Lem J, Krasnoperova NV, Calvert PD et al (1999) Morphological, physiological, and biochemical changes in rhodopsin knockout mice. Proc Natl Acad Sci U S A 96(2):736–741

Leonard KC, Petrin D, Coupland SG et al (2002) XIAP protection of photoreceptors in animal models of retinitis pigmentosa. PLoS One 2(3):e314

Léveillard T, Sahel JA (2010) Rod-derived cone viability factor for treating blinding diseases: from clinic to redox signaling. Sci Transl Med 2(26):26ps16

Léveillard T, Mohand-Said S, Lorentz O et al (2004) Identification and characterization of rod-derived cone viability factor. Nat Genet 36:755–759

Lewin AS, Drenser KA, Hauswirth WW et al (1998) Ribozyme rescue of photoreceptor cells in a transgenic rat model of autosomal dominant retinitis pigmentosa. Nat Med 4:967–971

Li Y, Tao W, Luo L, Huang D et al (2010) CNTF induces regeneration of cone outer segments in a rat model of retinal degeneration. PLoS One 5:e9495

Lima WF, Prakash TP, Murray HM et al (2012) Single-stranded siRNAs activate RNAi in animals. Cell 150(5):883–894

Littink KW, den Hollander A, Cremers FP, Collin RW (2012) The power of homozygosity mapping: discovery of new genetic defects in patients with retinal dystrophy. Adv Exp Med Biol 723:345–351

Liu J, Yu D, Aiba Y et al (2013) ss-siRNAs allele selectively inhibit ataxin-3 expression: multiple mechanisms for an alternative gene silencing strategy. Nucleic Acids Res 41(20):9570–9583

Low BE, Krebs MP, Joung JK et al (2014) Correction of the Crb1rd8 allele and retinal phenotype in C57BL/6 N mice via TALEN-mediated homology-directed repair. Invest Ophthalmol Vis Sci 55:387–395

Maclaren RE, Groppe M, Barnard AR et al (2014) Retinal gene therapy in patients with choroideremia: initial findings from a phase 1/2 clinical trial. Lancet 383(9923):1129–1137

Maguire AM, Simonelli F, Pierce EA et al (2008) Safety and efficacy of gene transfer for Leber's congenital amaurosis. N Engl J Med 358:2240–2248

Mao H, James T Jr, Schwein A et al (2011) AAV delivery of wild-type rhodopsin preserves retinal function in a mouse model of autosomal dominant retinitis pigmentosa. Hum Gene Ther 22:567–575

Mao H, Gorbatyuk MS, Rossmiller B, Hauswirth WW, Lewin AS (2012) Long-term rescue of retinal structure and function by rhodopsin RNA replacement with a single adeno-associated viral vector in P23H RHO transgenic mice. Hum Gene Ther 23(4):356–366

Marigo V (2007) Programmed cell death in retinal degeneration: targeting apoptosis in photoreceptors as potential therapy for retinal degeneration. Cell Cycle 6(6):652–655

McWilliam P, Farrar GJ, Kenna P et al (1989) Autosomal dominant retinitis pigmentosa (ADRP): localization of an ADRP gene to the long arm of chromosome 3. Genomics 5(3):619–622

Millington-Ward S, O'Neill B, Tuohy G et al (1997) Strategems in vitro for gene therapies directed to dominant mutations. Hum Mol Genet 6:1415–1426

Millington-Ward S, Chadderton N, O'Reilly M et al (2011) Suppression and replacement gene therapy for autosomal dominant disease in a murine model of dominant retinitis pigmentosa. Mol Ther 19:642–649

Miyagishi M, Hayashi M, Taira K (2003) Comparison of the suppressive effects of antisense oligonucleotides and siRNAs directed against the same targets in mammalian cells. Antisense Nucleic Acid Drug Dev 13:1–7

Mullard A (2011) Gene therapies advance towards finish line. Nat Rev Drug Discov 10:719–720

Mussolino C, Sanges D, Marrocco E et al (2011) Zinc-finger-based transcriptional repression of rhodopsin in a model of dominant retinitis pigmentosa. EMBO Mol Med 3:118–128

Nakazawa M (2011) Effects of calcium ion, calpains, and calcium channel blockers on retinitis pigmentosa. J Ophthalmol 2011:292040

Neveling K, Collin RW, Gilissen C et al (2012) Next-generation genetic testing for retinitis pigmentosa. Hum Mutat 33(6):963–972

Ohnaka M, Miki K, Gong YY et al (2012) Long-term expression of glial cell line-derived neurotrophic factor slows, but does not stop retinal degeneration in a model of retinitis pigmentosa. J Neurochem 122(5):1047–1053

O'Reilly M, Palfi A, Chadderton N et al (2007) RNA interference-mediated suppression and replacement of human rhodopsin in vivo. Am J Hum Genet 81:127–135

Ott J (1974) Estimate of the recombination fraction in human pedigrees: efficient computation of the likelihood of human linkage studies. Am J Hum Genet 26:588–597

Overlack N, Goldmann T, Wolfrum U et al (2012) Gene repair of an Usher syndrome causing mutation by zinc-finger nuclease mediated homologous recombination. Invest Ophthalmol Vis Sci 53:4140–4146

Palfi A, Ader M, Kiang AS et al (2006) RNAi-based suppression and replacement of RDS-peripherin in retinal organotypic culture. Hum Mutat 27:260–268

Palfi A, Millington-Ward S, Chadderton N et al (2010) Adeno-associated virus-mediated rhodopsin replacement provides therapeutic benefit in mice with a targeted disruption of the rhodopsin gene. Hum Gene Ther 21:311–323

Palfi A, Chadderton N, McKee AG et al (2012) Efficacy of codelivery of dual AAV2/5 vectors in the murine retina and hippocampus. Hum Gene Ther 23:847–858

Perche O, Doly M, Ranchon-Cole I (2007) Caspase-dependent apoptosis in light-induced retinal degeneration. Invest Ophthalmol Vis Sci 48(6):2753–2759

Petrs-Silva H, Yasumura D, Matthes MT et al (2012) Suppression of rds expression by siRNA and gene replacement strategies for gene therapy using rAAV vector. Adv Exp Med Biol 723:215–223

Ratnapriya R, Swaroop A (2013) Genetic architecture of retinal and macular degenerative diseases: the promise and challenges of next-generation sequencing. Genome Med 5:84

Sakami S, Maeda T, Bereta G et al (2011) Probing mechanisms of photoreceptor degeneration in a new mouse model of the common form of autosomal dominant retinitis pigmentosa due to P23H opsin mutations. J Biol Chem 286:10551–10567

Sano Y, Furuta A, Setsuie R et al (2006) Photoreceptor cell apoptosis in the retinal degeneration of Uchl3-deficient mice. Am J Pathol 169(1):132–141

Schlichtenbrede FC, da Cruz L, Stephens C et al (2003) Long-term evaluation of retinal function in Prph2Rd2/Rd2 mice following AAV-mediated gene replacement therapy. J Gene Med 5(9):757–764

Schwahn U, Lenzner S, Dong J et al (1998) Positional cloning of the gene ofr X-linked retinitis pigmentosa 2. Nat Genet 19:327

Schweiger MR, Kerick M, Timmermann B et al (2009) Genome-wide massively parallel sequencing of form-aldehyde fixed-paraffin embedded (FFPE) tumor tissues for copy-number- and mutation-analysis. PLoS One 4(5):e5548

Shanks ME, Downes SM, Copley RR et al (2013) Next-generation sequencing (NGS) as a diagnostic tool for retinal degeneration reveals a much higher detection rate in early-onset disease. Eur J Hum Genet 21(3):274–280

Singh G, Lott MT, Wallace DC (1989) A mitochondrial DNA mutation as a cause of Leber's hereditary optic neuropathy. N Engl J Med 320:1300–1305

Sung CH, Davenport CM, Hennessy JC (1991) Rhodopsin mutations in autosomal dominant retinitis pigmentosa. Proc Natl Acad Sci U S A 88:6481–6485

Tam LC, Kiang AS, Kennan A et al (2008) Therapeutic benefit derived from RNAi-mediated ablation of IMPDH1 transcripts in a murine model of autosomal dominant retinitis pigmentosa (RP10). Hum Mol Genet 17:2084–2100

Tam LC, Kiang AS, Campbell M et al (2010) Prevention of autosomal dominant retinitis pigmentosa by systemic drug therapy targeting heat shock protein 90 (Hsp90). Hum Mol Genet 19:4421–4436

Tijsterman M, Plasterk RH (2004) Dicers at RISC; the mechanism of RNAi. Cell 117:1–3

Touchard E, Heiduschka P, Berdugo M et al (2012) Non-viral gene therapy for GDNF production in RCS rat: the crucial role of the plasmid dose. Gene Ther 19:886–898

Trapani I, Colella P, Sommella A et al (2014) Effective delivery of large genes to the retina by dual AAV vectors. EMBO Mol Med 6:194–211

Trifunović D, Sahaboglu A, Kaur J, Mencl S, Zrenner E, Ueffing M, Arango-Gonzalez B, Paquet-Durand F (2012) Neuroprotective strategies for the treatment of inherited photoreceptor degeneration. Curr Mol Med 12(5):598–612

Usui S, Oveson BC, Lee SY et al (2009) NADPH oxidase plays a central role in cone cell death in retinitis pigmentosa. J Neurochem 110:1028–1037

Usui S, Oveson BC, Iwase T et al (2011) Overexpression of SOD in retina: need for increase in H_2O_2-detoxifying enzyme in same cellular compartment. Free Radic Biol Med 51:1347–1354

Vandenberghe LH, Bell P, Maguire AM et al (2013) AAV9 targets cone photoreceptors in the nonhuman primate retina. PLoS One 8:e353263

Van den Heuvel DM, Harschnitz O, van den Berg LH et al (2014) Taking a risk: a therapeutic focus on ataxin-2 in amyotrophic lateral sclerosis? Trends Mol Med 20:25–35

Wallace DC, Singh G, Lott MT et al (1988) Mitochondrial DNA mutation associated with Leber's hereditary optic neuropathy. Science 242:1427–1430

Xia H, Mao Q, Eliason SL et al (2004) RNAi suppresses polyglutamine-induced neurodegeneration in a model of spinocerebellar ataxia. Nat Med 10:816–820

Yang Y, Mohand-Said S, Danan A et al (2009) Functional cone rescue by RdCVF protein in a dominant model of retinitis pigmentosa. Mol Ther 17:787–795

Yao J, Jia L, Khan N, Zheng QD, Moncrief A, Hauswirth WW, Thompson DA, Zacks DN (2012) Caspase inhibition with XIAP as an adjunct to AAV vector gene-replacement therapy: improving efficacy and prolonging the treatment window. PLoS One 7(5):e37197

Zamore PD, Tuschl T, Sharp PA, Bartel DP (2000) RNAi: double-stranded RNA directs the ATP-dependent cleavage of mRNA at 21 to 23 nucleotide intervals. Cell 101(1):25–33

Zaneveld J, Wang F, Wang X, Chen R (2013) Dawn of ocular gene therapy: implications for molecular diagnosis in retinal disease. Sci China Life Sci 56(2):125–133

Age-Related Macular Degeneration: The Challenges

Elizabeth P. Rakoczy, Cecinio C. Ronquillo Jr.,
Samuel F. Passi, Balamurali K. Ambati, Aaron Nagiel,
Robert Lanza, and Steven D. Schwartz

Age related macular degeneration (AMD or ARMD) is the most common cause of vision loss in the developed world (Mitchell et al. 1995; Friedman et al. 2004a). Almost two million people in the United States have AMD, and the prevalence of the disease is expected to jump almost twofold from 1.75 million in 2000 to 2.95 million in 2020 (Friedman et al. 2004b). The prevalence of AMD rises from 0.7 % in the 65–74 years age group to 5.4 % in the 75–84 years age group and to 18.5 % in people over 85 (Mitchell et al. 1995). As a result of population aging, the number of people with AMD is likely to increase substantially worldwide over the next decade.

AMD is a degenerative condition that affects the macula, a small area in the central retina that is responsible for 80 % of human visual activities, including high-acuity vision and reading. AMD has many nuanced phenotypes but is typically lumped into two clinical presentations, each with distinct treatment and prognostic ramifications.

The non-exudative, atrophic, or dry form of AMD is associated with retinal pigment epithelium (RPE) abnormalities and can culminate in widespread loss of macular structures. The atrophic loss of the RPE and subsequently the photoreceptors and choriocapillaris has come to be known as geographic atrophy (GA). This form of the disease is associated with gradual vision loss and affects approximately 85 % of AMD sufferers. The clinical course and pathogenesis of dry-AMD are intimately related to the health of the RPE monolayer. The RPE serves several essential functions in the retina, including the phagocytosis of photoreceptor outer segments, the formation of the blood-retina barrier, and the maintenance of ionic and metabolic homeostasis (Zarbin 2004).

E.P. Rakoczy, PhD (✉)
Department of Molecular Ophthalmology, Centre for Ophthalmology and Visual Sciences, The University of Western Australia, Crawley, WA, Australia
e-mail: elizabeth.rakoczy@uwa.edu.au

C.C. Ronquillo Jr., PhD • S.F. Passi, BA
Department of Ophthalmology and Visual Sciences, University of Utah School of Medicine, John A. Moran Eye Center, University of Utah Health Sciences Center, Salt Lake City, UT, USA
e-mail: nikko.ronquillo@hsc.utah.edu; samuel.passi@hsc.utah.edu

B.K. Ambati, MD, PhD, MBA
Department of Ophthalmology, University of Utah, Salt Lake City, UT, USA
e-mail: bala.ambati@utah.edu

A. Nagiel, MD, PhD
Department of Ophthalmology, University of California, Los Angeles, CA, USA
e-mail: nagiel@jsei.ucla.edu

R. Lanza, MD
Advanced Cell Technology, Marlborough, Massachusetts, USA
e-mail: rlanza@advancedcell.com

S.D. Schwartz, MD
Retina Division, Jules Stein Eye Institute, David Geffen School of Medicine, University of California, Los Angeles, Los Angeles, CA, USA
e-mail: Schwartz@jsei.ucla.edu

The earliest pathogenic step in dry-AMD is thought to be oxidative stress of the RPE owing to the accumulation of lipofuscin and breakdown products of retinaldehyde (Shen et al. 2007). The accumulation of toxic metabolites such as A2E within RPE cells eventually leads to RPE apoptosis and resultant GA. The underlying degenerative process is not entirely clear and may involve choroidal ischemia (Coleman et al. 2013), but regardless, AMD pathogenesis is multifactorial with many genetic and environmental influences, including diet and smoking (Ratnapriya and Chew 2013). Genome-wide association studies have established a strong link between AMD and the complement pathway, but how dysregulation of complement factors leads to GA is being explored (Anderson et al. 2010; Zhou et al. 2006).

The treatment options for dry-AMD remain limited. The only widely accepted intervention in patients with dry-AMD has been a specific combination of antioxidants established by the Age-Related Eye Disease Study (Age-Related Eye Disease Study Research 2001). Designed with the intent to treat the underlying oxidative stress, this AREDS formula showed modest benefit in reducing the risk of progression from intermediate AMD to advanced AMD, which includes central GA and wet-AMD. The recently completed AREDS 2 trial (Age-Related Eye Disease Study 2 Research 2013) attempted to refine the hypothesis of AREDS, but the results did not meet statistical significance. As of yet, there is no well-established treatment to slow the progression of GA. No treatment exists that reverses the visual losses suffered with dry-AMD. Several drug classes are being tested in early clinical trials, including neuroprotectants, visual cycle modulators, immunosuppressants, and complement factor pathway inhibitors (Damico et al. 2012).

The exudative, neovascular, or wet form of AMD is defined by the presence of choroidal neovascularization. The exudative form is more aggressive and is responsible for 90 % of cases of severe vision loss. Wet-AMD occurs when retinal pigment epithelium (RPE) cells fail to stop the choroidal blood vessels from growing into the retina (Ambati and Fowler 2012). When these capillaries enter the retina, they grow rapidly, resulting in fluid and blood leaking into the retina (Fig. 5.1). Although the wet form of AMD can lead to more sudden and progressive visual loss due to hemorrhage, fluid exudation, and eventual scarring, its treatment has been revolutionized by the use of anti-vascular endothelial growth factor (VEGF) agents.

There are several factors understood to be involved in angiogenesis in the eye, with vascular endothelial growth factor (VEGF) playing a central role. The VEGF protein is considered the most proximal to induction of angiogenesis, and it is involved in the underlying etiology of wet-AMD. The stimulus for upregulation of VEGF in AMD is thought to be hypoxia and/or inflammation. In wet-AMD, VEGF has been reported to be present below the RPE cell layer and around photoreceptors (Kwak et al. 2000). The involvement of pigment epithelial-derived factor (PEDF) in CNV development is less well understood. PEDF is a serine protease inhibitor reported to inhibit angiogenesis in the retina (Dawson et al. 1999; Stellmach et al. 2001). In addition, complement factors B and H have also been linked to the development of wet-AMD. Evidence of this comes from genetic analyses of patients with wet-AMD (Hageman et al. 2005). The complement cascade normally protects the body against invading bacteria, but if the pathway is overactive, the cascade may induce inflammation leading to tissue damage (Marx 2006).

To date, blocking the VEGF pathway has been the most beneficial method for inhibiting neovascular growth (Kaiser 2006). Recently, therapies using recombinant humanized anti-VEGF antibody fragments or soluble receptor decoys (e.g., ranibizumab [Lucentis®], bevacizumab [Avastin®], aflibercept [Eylea®] (Mousa and Mousa 2010)) have shown that wet-AMD can be treated successfully. However, these therapies do not address the underlying cause of the development of wet-AMD, and the patients require frequent ocular injections at 4–8-week intervals which is inconvenient, associated with cumulative risks of repeated injections, and very expensive (Steinbrook 2006). Thus, there remains a need for the development of novel strategies for sustained and efficient drug delivery into the eye of wet-AMD patients.

Fig. 5.1 Graphical presentation of wet-AMD or wet-ARMD

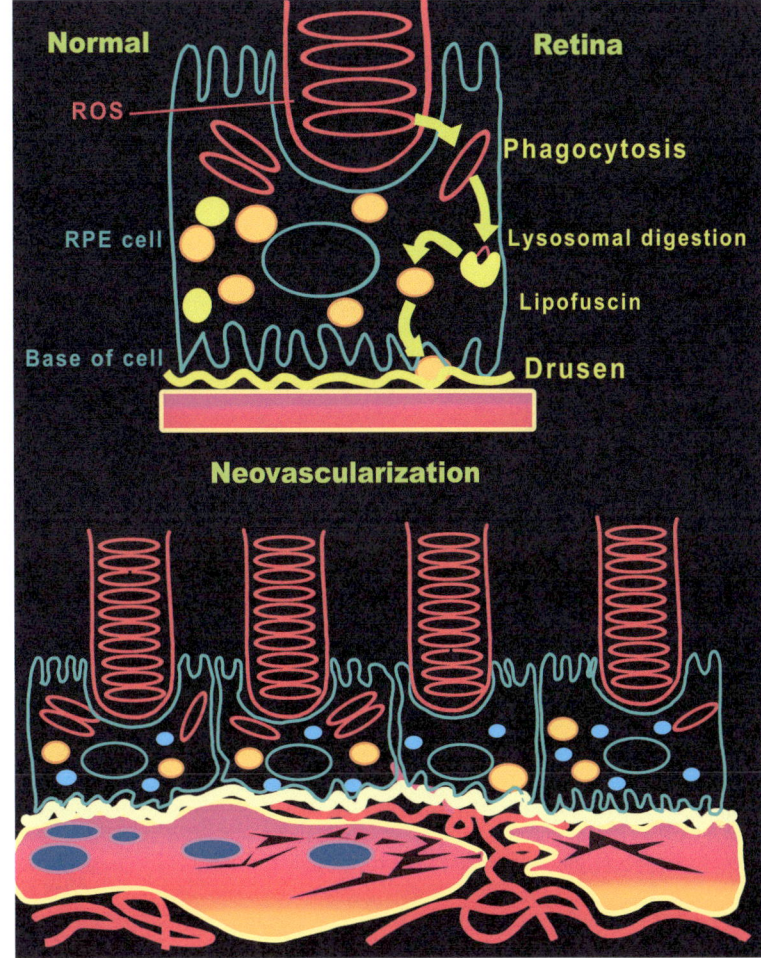

The dream of every ARMD geneticist is that one or more of the genes that have been identified from family-based or case control association studies will prove to be a suitable target for a definitive therapy to block the development of ARMD or to arrest its progression. However, as we learn more about this complex genetic disorder, many of us are coming to realize that, with the exception of a relatively small number of individuals and families who develop their ARMD as a result of a highly penetrant and rare genetic variant (such as the one described recently by (Raychaudhuri et al. 2011) for CFH), we cannot view the treatment of ARMD in the same fashion that we would think of a monogenic disorder in which a single genetic lesion is causative of disease. To date, the effects of the multiple genes that have been implicated in ARMD incidence and/or progression act predominantly in an additive fashion suggesting that each genetic variant contributes independently to the overall risk to the individual. In practical terms, we do not know if the future therapy for ARMD will be multifactorial and potentially involve a combination of diet, lifestyle and pharmacologic interventions or if we will be able to have a major impact on the disease condition, despite its diverse genetic and non-genetic contributors, by acting upon a single pathway (Gorin 2012).

Compliance with Ethical Requirements E.P. Rakoczy, C.C. Ronquillo, S.F. Passi, B.K. Ambati, Aaron Nagiel, Robert Lanza, and Steven D. Schwartz declare that they have no conflict of interest.

No human or animal studies were carried out for this chapter.

References

Age-Related Eye Disease Study Research G (2001) A randomized, placebo-controlled, clinical trial of high-dose supplementation with vitamins C and E, beta carotene, and zinc for age-related macular degeneration and vision loss: AREDS report no. 8. Arch Ophthalmol 119(10):1417–1436

Age-Related Eye Disease Study 2 Research G (2013) Lutein + zeaxanthin and omega-3 fatty acids for age-related macular degeneration: the Age-Related Eye Disease Study 2 (AREDS2) randomized clinical trial. JAMA 309(19):2005–2015. doi:10.1001/jama.2013.4997

Ambati J, Fowler BJ (2012) Mechanisms of age-related macular degeneration. Neuron 75(1):26–39. doi:10.1016/j.neuron.2012.06.018

Anderson DH, Radeke MJ, Gallo NB, Chapin EA, Johnson PT, Curletti CR, Hancox LS, Hu J, Ebright JN, Malek G, Hauser MA, Rickman CB, Bok D, Hageman GS, Johnson LV (2010) The pivotal role of the complement system in aging and age-related macular degeneration: hypothesis re-visited. Prog Retin Eye Res 29(2):95–9112

Coleman DJ, Silverman RH, Rondeau MJ, Lloyd HO, Khanifar AA, Chan RV (2013) Age-related macular degeneration: choroidal ischaemia? Br J Ophthalmol 97(8):1020–1023. doi:10.1136/bjophthalmol-2013-303143

Damico FM, Gasparin F, Scolari MR, Pedral LS, Takahashi BS (2012) New approaches and potential treatments for dry age-related macular degeneration. Arq Bras Oftalmol 75(1):71–76

Dawson DW, Volpert OV, Gillis P, Crawford SE, Xu H, Benedict W, Bouck NP (1999) Pigment epithelium-derived factor: a potent inhibitor of angiogenesis. Science 285(5425):245–248

Friedman DS, O'Colmain BJ, Munoz B, Tomany SC, McCarty C, de Jong PT, Nemesure B, Mitchell P, Kempen J (2004a) Prevalence of age-related macular degeneration in the United States. Arch Ophthalmol 122(4):564–572. doi:10.1001/archopht.122.4.564

Friedman DS, O'Colmain BJ, Munoz B, Tomany SC, McCarty C, de Jong PT, Nemesure B, Mitchell P, Kempen J, Eye Diseases Prevalence Research G (2004b) Prevalence of age-related macular degeneration in the United States. Arch Ophthalmol 122(4):564–572. doi:10.1001/archopht.122.4.564

Gorin MB (2012) Genetic insights into age-related macular degeneration: controversies addressing risk, causality, and therapeutics. Mol Aspects Med 33(4):467–486. http://dx.doi.org/10.1016/j.mam.2012.04.004

Hageman GS, Anderson DH, Johnson LV, Hancox LS, Taiber AJ, Hardisty LI, Hageman JL, Stockman HA, Borchardt JD, Gehrs KM, Smith RJ, Silvestri G, Russell SR, Klaver CC, Barbazetto I, Chang S, Yannuzzi LA, Barile GR, Merriam JC, Smith RT, Olsh AK, Bergeron J, Zernant J, Merriam JE, Gold B, Dean M, Allikmets R (2005) A common haplotype in the complement regulatory gene factor H (HF1/CFH) predisposes individuals to age-related macular degeneration. Proc Natl Acad Sci U S A 102(20):7227–7232. doi:10.1073/pnas.0501536102

Kaiser PK (2006) Antivascular endothelial growth factor agents and their development: therapeutic implications in ocular diseases. Am J Ophthalmol 142(4):660–668. doi:10.1016/j.ajo.2006.05.061

Kwak N, Okamoto N, Wood JM, Campochiaro PA (2000) VEGF is major stimulator in model of choroidal neovascularization. Invest Ophthalmol Vis Sci 41(10):3158–3164

Marx J (2006) Genetics – a clearer view of macular degeneration. Science 311(5768):1704–1705. doi:10.1126/science.311.5768.1704

Mitchell P, Smith W, Attebo K, Wang JJ (1995) Prevalence of age-related maculopathy in Australia. The Blue Mountains Eye Study. Ophthalmology 102(10):1450–1460

Mousa SA, Mousa SS (2010) Current status of vascular endothelial growth factor inhibition in age-related macular degeneration. BioDrugs 24(3):183–194. doi:10.2165/11318550-000000000-00000

Ratnapriya R, Chew EY (2013) Age-related macular degeneration-clinical review and genetics update. Clin Genet 84(2):160–166. doi:10.1111/cge.12206

Raychaudhuri S, Iartchouk O, Chin K, Tan PL, Tai AK, Ripke S, Gowrisankar S, Vemuri S, Montgomery K, Yu Y, Reynolds R, Zack DJ, Campochiaro B, Campochiaro P, Katsanis N, Daly MJ, Seddon JM (2011) A rare penetrant mutation in CFH confers high risk of age-related macular degeneration. Nat Genet 43(12):1232–U1291. doi:10.1038/Ng.976

Shen JK, Dong A, Hackett SF, Bell WR, Green WR, Campochiaro PA (2007) Oxidative damage in age-related macular degeneration. Histol Histopathol 22(12):1301–1308

Steinbrook R (2006) The price of sight–ranibizumab, bevacizumab, and the treatment of macular degeneration. N Engl J Med 355(14):1409–1412. doi:10.1056/NEJMp068185

Stellmach V, Crawford SE, Zhou W, Bouck N (2001) Prevention of ischemia-induced retinopathy by the natural ocular antiangiogenic agent pigment epithelium-derived factor. Proc Natl Acad Sci U S A 98(5):2593–2597. doi:10.1073/pnas.031252398

Zarbin MA (2004) Current concepts in the pathogenesis of age-related macular degeneration. Arch Ophthalmol 122(4):598–614

Zhou J, Jang YP, Kim SR, Sparrow JR (2006) Complement activation by photooxidation products of A2E, a lipofuscin constituent of the retinal pigment epithelium. Proc Natl Acad Sci U S A 103(44):16182–16187

Neovascular Age-Related Macular Degeneration: Secretion Gene Therapy

Elizabeth P. Rakoczy, Chooi-May Lai, and Ian J. Constable

6.1 The Road to Gene Therapy Treatment of a Complex Disease, Wet-ARMD

The Department of Molecular Ophthalmology at the Lions Eye Institute, Perth, was founded in 1989 with the aim of using technological breakthroughs for the treatment of blindness. We began studying a new technology based on recombinant adeno-associated virus (rAAV) vector, initially targeting a rare monogenic disease known as Leber's congenital amaurosis (LCA). By 2000, in collaboration with Prof Kristina Narfstrom, we injected 12 Briard dogs (an excellent model for LCA) with rAAV carrying the RPE65 gene and confirmed the remarkable improvement in vision, earlier published by the Bennett Lab (Acland et al. 2001). This work gave us a very useful insight into the power and longevity of gene therapy. Encouraged by its promise (Narfstrom et al. 2003a, b), we decided to apply our learnings toward preclinical development of rAAV gene therapy for a more common disease: wet-ARMD or wet-AMD.

6.2 Major Milestones (See Table 6.1)

Initial studies demonstrated that hypoxia and/or inflammation induced the enhanced production of Vascular Endothelial Growth Factor (VEGF) in a wide variety of retinal cells, leading to neovascularization (Sandercoe et al. 2003). Because the source and timing of VEGF production remained unknown, attempting to downregulate VEGF by targeting the source was not a feasible strategy. Complicating matters, several human isoforms of VEGF were identified, including isoforms 206, 189, 183, 165, 148, 145, and 121 (Wulff et al. 2001; Ferrara 2004). Therefore, it seemed likely that the most effective treatment would neutralize all isoforms of excess VEGF, regardless of their origin.

Our goal was to achieve long-term delivery of a therapeutic agent with a single injection. We recognized that the rAAV system was well suited for that purpose, as animal studies demonstrated that AAV-mediated transgene expression could last for several years (Bennett et al. 1999; Narfstrom et al. 2008). We developed the concept of *secretion gene therapy* (Lai et al. 2002), which

E.P. Rakoczy, PhD (✉) • C.-M. Lai, PhD
Department of Molecular Ophthalmology,
Centre for Ophthalmology and Visual Sciences,
The University of Western Australia,
Crawley, WA, Australia
e-mail: elizabeth.rakoczy@uwa.edu.au;
may.lai@uwa.edu.au

I.J. Constable, MBBS, DSc, FRANZCO
Department of Ophthalmology, Lions Eye Institute,
Sir Charles Gairdner Hospital, University of
Western Australia, Crawley, WA, Australia
e-mail: Ian.Constable@lei.org.au

E.P. Rakoczy (ed.), *Gene- and Cell-Based Treatment Strategies for the Eye*, Essentials in Ophthalmology,
DOI 10.1007/978-3-662-45188-5_6, © Springer-Verlag Berlin Heidelberg 2015

Table 6.1 Experimental completion and publication time line

Year of completion	Experimental milestone	Publication
1998	Selection of rAAV as a suitable delivery vehicle	Rolling et al. (1999)
2000	Selection of sFlt-1 as the transgene (neovascular inhibitor)	Lai et al. (2001)
2002	Efficacy of rAAV.sFlt-1 in transient neovascular models	Lai et al. (2002)
2003	Laser model for CNV in the monkey	Shen et al. (2004)
2004	Establishment of long-term mouse model (Kimba)	Lai et al. (2005a)
2005	Long-term efficacy of rAAV.sFlt-1 in Kimba mice	Lai et al. (2005b)
2007	Immunological safety of rAAV.sFlt-1 in mice	Lai et al. (2009)
2008	rAAV.sFlt-1 preclinical safety in monkeys	Lai et al. (2012)
2012	Start of Phase I/IIa clinical trial in humans	

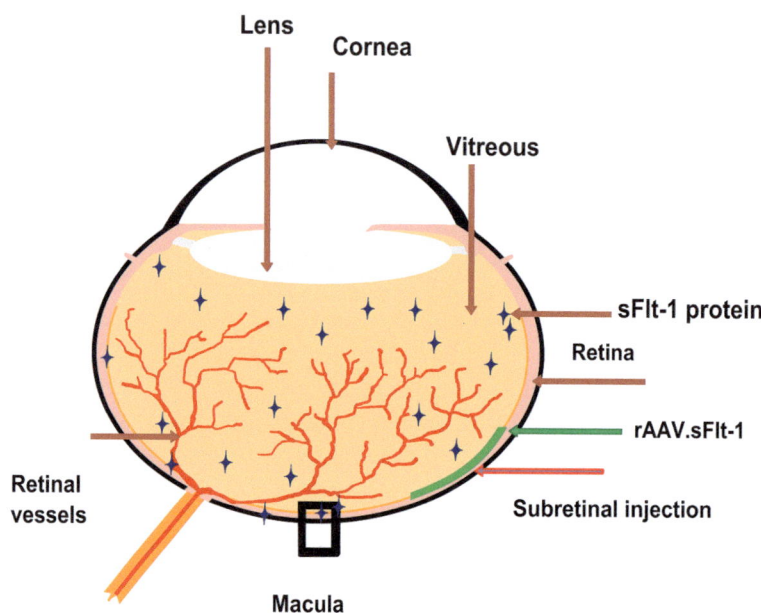

Fig. 6.1 Graphical presentation of the concept of secretion gene therapy

differs from traditional gene therapy in several ways. Unlike gene therapy for monogenic diseases, it does not aim to correct a specific mutation or even target the diseased cells; instead, it produces a soluble protein in the proximity of the abnormal cells, which acts as a drug that interferes with the disease pathway (Fig. 6.1).

6.2.1 Selection of the Transgene

For the selection of the transgene, we evaluated candidates based on multiple criteria: (1) a transgene had to be non-toxic, (2) non-immunogenic, (3) could be inserted into the rAAV (<4.5 kb), (4) could be secreted by the host cells, and (5) was small enough to be distributed across the retina by diffusion and natural fluid movement.

The existence of VEGF as the driving force behind neovascularization necessary for solid cancer growth was first hypothesized in 1971 by Prof Judah Folkman (Folkman et al. 1971). The idea struggled to gain acceptance in the scientific community; only following the cloning of the VEGF gene (Leung et al. 1989) did a series of studies confirm the role of VEGF in cancer development as well as several ocular neovascular diseases including diabetic retinopathy (Adamis et al. 1994), wet-ARMD (Churchill et al. 2006), and corneal vascularization (Amano et al. 1998). In 1990, Genentech initiated clinical trials on the first anti-VEGF compound, a VEGF-antibody, demonstrating that excess VEGF trapping is an efficient way of inhibiting neovascularization. By this time, there was an increasing amount of data suggesting that the long-term neutralization of excess VEGF in the eyes of patients suffering from wet-ARMD would be beneficial for improving their vision (Trujillo et al. 2007). Although the eye is considered to be an immune-privileged organ, one of the major challenges of protein-based therapies is to deal with the potential immune reaction. Thus, we decided to focus our search for an antiangiogenic agent among natural products.

Data from animal studies (Shen et al. 1998; Lai et al. 2005a) demonstrated that retinal/choroidal neovascularization was closely associated with the presence of elevated levels of VEGF in the eye. VEGF is a secreted protein that migrates to its receptors on the endothelial cells. VEGF exerts its action via specific *fms*-like receptors, Flt-1 (VEGF-R1) and Flk-1/KDR (VEGFR2), which are high-affinity receptor tyrosine kinases (de Vries et al. 1992). Both are membrane-spanning receptors that contain seven immunoglobulin-like domains in the extracellular ligand-binding region and cytoplasmic tyrosine-kinase domains (de Vries et al. 1992). The soluble truncated form of the VEGF receptor 1, sFlt-1, is the only known endogenous, specific inhibitor of VEGF. sFlt-1 is generated by alternative splicing and lacks the membrane-proximal immunoglobulin-like domain, the transmembrane-spanning region, and the intracellular tyrosine-kinase domain. sFlt-1 is generated by alternative splicing and acts as a potent VEGF antagonist either through high-affinity binding and sequestration of VEGF, to which it binds with high affinity, or through forming inactive heterodimers with membrane-spanning isoforms of the VEGF receptors Flt-1 and KDR (Kendall and Thomas 1993; Kendall et al. 1996). Although sFlt-1 binds to VEGF with the same affinity and specificity as the full-length receptor, the binding does not initiate signal transduction (Kendall et al. 1996; Barleon et al. 1997).

These favorable characteristics of sFlt-1 have attracted considerable attention for its potential clinical application in the inhibition of angiogenesis (Kendall and Thomas 1993; Goldman et al. 1998; Kong et al. 1998). As sFlt-1 is endogenously expressed (i.e., is a self-antigen), exogenous sFlt-1 would not be recognized as a foreign antigen. The efficacy of sFlt-1 in terms of VEGF binding and inhibition of neovascularization had been demonstrated (Kendall and Thomas 1993). On the basis of these publications and our preliminary data (Lai et al. 2001), *we selected sFlt-1 as the transgene to begin preclinical development for wet-ARMD.*

6.2.2 Selection of the Delivery Vector

Several viral vector systems were available for the transduction of postmitotic somatic cells, including lentiviral, adenoviral, and AAV vector systems. Unlike other viral vector systems, the AAV vector was derived from a nonpathogenic, conditionally replicating wild-type virus. In preclinical studies, ocular administration of rAAV vectors was associated with minimal toxicity and immunogenicity. These favorable characteristics made AAV an ideal candidate for use in gene therapy to treat ocular diseases. rAAV vector had been tested extensively in animals for gene transfer, transgene expression, and target specificity in the eye. In rodent models, a serotype 2 AAV vector encoding the reporter gene green fluorescent protein (GFP) under the control of the ubiquitous CMV promoter was shown to primarily transduce photoreceptors and RPE cells following subretinal injection (Auricchio et al. 2001). In rats and monkeys, which possess very similar retinal-choroid circulation and macular anatomy to the human eye, subretinal administration of rAAV.GFP resulted in efficient and stable transduction of photoreceptors and RPE cells (Bennett et al. 1999; Rolling et al. 1999, 2000). *On this basis we selected rAAV(2) as our delivery system for wet-AMD gene therapy.*

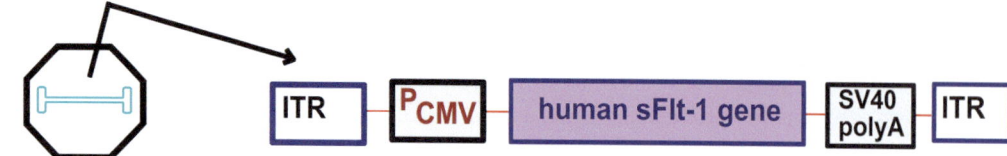

rAAV.CMV.sFlt-1

Fig. 6.2 Plasmid map of the rAAV.CMV.sFlt-1 vector

6.2.3 The Construct

6.2.3.1 Construction of the Vector Plasmid pAAV.CMV.sFlt-1

The sFlt-1 fragment was subcloned into plasmid pCI which contained the cytomegalovirus (CMV) major immediate-early gene enhancer/promoter, a chimeric intron, and a simian virus 40 polyadenylation (SV40 polyA) signal. The resultant CMV-sFlt-1-SV40 polyA construct was then cloned into AAV plasmid SSV9 (psub201); (Samulski et al. 1989) to generate the rAAV.CMV.sFlt-1 vector (Fig. 6.2).

6.2.4 In Vitro Data

The transduction efficiency of and sFlt-1 protein production by rAAV.CMV.sFlt-1 was tested in vitro in a variety of human cell lines. The human RPE cells ARPE19 and D407 were particularly amenable to rAAV transduction (data not shown). We also tested sFlt-1 protein production in hRPE51 cells and in HEK-293 cells. In addition, the efficacy of the sFlt-1 protein produced was tested for its ability to inhibit VEGF-driven proliferation of human umbilical vein endothelial cells (HUVEC) (Fig. 6.3).

6.2.5 Preclinical Data

Five preclinical studies have been conducted using the rAAV.sFlt-1 vector in animal models of ocular neovascularization (Lai et al. 2002, 2005b, 2009, 2012). These studies were conducted on the Kimba transgenic mice and the laser model of

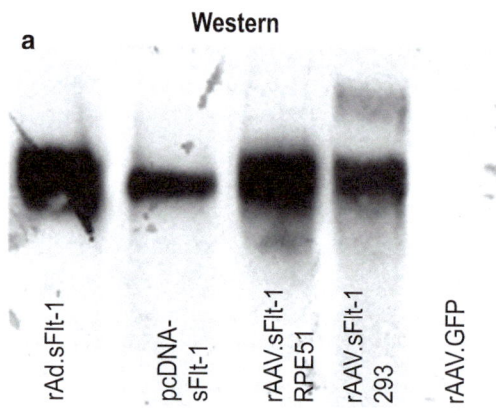

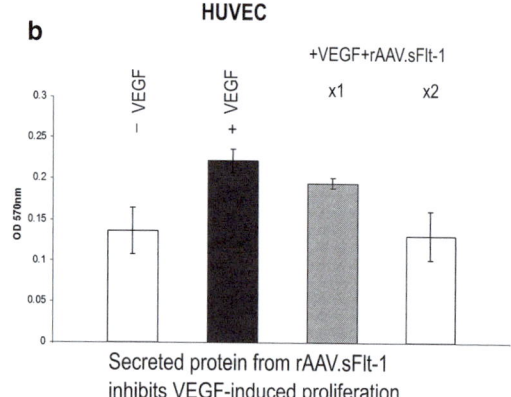

Fig. 6.3 Demonstration of sFlt-1 protein production and efficacy test. (**a**) Western blot showing presence of sFlt-1 protein in supernatant from RPE51 cells transduced with a recombinant adenovirus (Lane 1), transfected with pcDNA.sFlt-1 DNA (Lane 2), transduced with rAAV.sFlt-1 (Lane 3) or rAAV.GFP (Lane 5). Lane 4 demonstrates sFlt-1 production in HK293 cells. (**b**) Graph showing the relative proliferation of HUVEC cells in the absence of VEGF (Lane 1), presence of VEGF (Lane 2), and presence of VEGF plus 1 μL (Lane 3) or 2 μL (Lane 4) conditioned media from rAAV.sFlt-1-transduced RPE51 cells

Table 6.2 Preclinical studies completed with the rAAV.sFlt-1 vector

Animal model	Number of rAAV. sFlt-1-injected animals	Dose administered (viral particles)	Reference
Kimba transgenic mice	13	1×10^{11}	Lai et al. (2005b)
Kimba transgenic mice	50	8×10^{9}	Lai et al. (2009)
Rats	32	8×10^{8}	Lai et al. (2002)
Macaque monkeys	5	4×10^{12}	Lai et al. (2005b)
Macaque monkeys	5	8×10^{11}	Lai et al. (2012)
Total treated animals	105		

choroidal neovascularization (CNV) using rats and macaque monkeys. Table 6.2 shows preclinical studies completed with the rAAV.sFlt-1 vector.

6.2.5.1 rAAV.sFlt-1 Studies in the Kimba Mice

Kimba mice with chronic, progressive retinal neovascularization and degeneration were used as an animal model (Lai et al. 2005a; Tee et al. 2008; Rakoczy et al. 2010; Ali Rahman et al. 2011; Vagaja et al. 2012; Binz et al. 2013) in two separate studies. In the first study, transgenic mice were assessed for ocular neovascular changes before and after administration of the rAAV. sFlt-1 vector (1×10^{11} viral particles) in one eye and control vector in the contralateral eye (Lai et al. 2005b). The eye injected with rAAV.sFlt-1 showed a statistically significant overall reduction in the neovascular grading from a median grade of "3" (before injection) to a median grade of "1" at 1 month after injection. This reduction was maintained at 3 and 8 months postinjection (Fig. 6.4).

The principal aim of the second study was to determine whether subretinal injection of rAAV. sFlt-1 resulted in any cell-mediated immune responses that could negatively impact long-term expression of sFlt-1 or cause immune response-associated damage to the retina (Lai et al. 2009). In this study, Kimba transgenic mice were given sub-retinal injections of rAAV.sFlt-1 in one eye and phosphate-buffered saline in the contralateral eye. Flow cytometric examination of the posterior eye cup showed that at 1 week postinjection, there was a localized, transient increase in CD45+ leucocytes and CD11b+ macrophages, but no differences in CD19+, CD8+, and CD4+ (B and T lymphocytes).

At 1 month postinjection, there was no difference detected in any of the leukocyte subsets (i.e., CD45+, CD19+, CD11b+, CD8+, or CD4+ cells). Flow cytometric evaluation of lymphocyte subsets of the spleens from these mice at the 1-week and 1-month time points showed no significant differences in the numbers of lymphocytes. This finding suggested that there was no systemic immune response present (Lai et al. 2009).

6.2.5.2 rAAV.sFlt-1 Study in Monkeys

The efficacy and safety of rAAV.sFlt-1 was also examined in a non-human primate (macaque) model of ARMD in which laser photocoagulation was used to induce CNV (Lai et al. 2005b). The retinal-choroid circulation and macular anatomy of macaques are very similar to that of the human, making them an ideal model for the investigation of the effect of sFlt-1 on CNV. In the first study on non-human primates, macaque monkeys were injected subretinally with rAAV. sFlt-1 in one eye and a control vector in the contralateral eye. Ocular assessments were conducted periodically after subretinal injection. No complications related to subretinal injection were apparent in either the control-injected or rAAV. sFlt-1-injected animals. To assess the long-term therapeutic efficacy of rAAV.sFlt-1, the injected monkeys were subjected to retinal laser injury to test whether CNV could be induced 16 months later. Eight laser lesions were delivered to each eye, and the eyes were monitored for development of CNV 2 and 4 weeks following laser injury. Whereas the control eyes developed CNV-related lesions, no CNV developed in the rAAV. sFlt-1-injected eyes.

Fig. 6.4 Fluorescein angiography images of Kimba eyes prior to injection (**a**, **b**); at 1 month postinjection (**c**, **d**) and at 8 months postinjection (**e**, **f**). *Arrowheads* demarcate boundary of bleb formed following subretinal injection. Histological images showing complete loss of photoreceptors in the atrophied retina of an eye injected with rAAV.GFP (**g**) and presence of aberrant blood vessels (arrows) in an eye (**h**) injected with rAAV. sFlt-1 at 8 months postinjection. Note the disappearance of white spots, signs of leakiness, in panel (**d**) and the presence of sclerotic vessels and the *gray color* of the atrophic retina (**e**) in the rAAV.GFP-injected eye. *INL* inner nuclear layer, *NFL* nerve fibre layer, *ONL* outer nuclear layer.

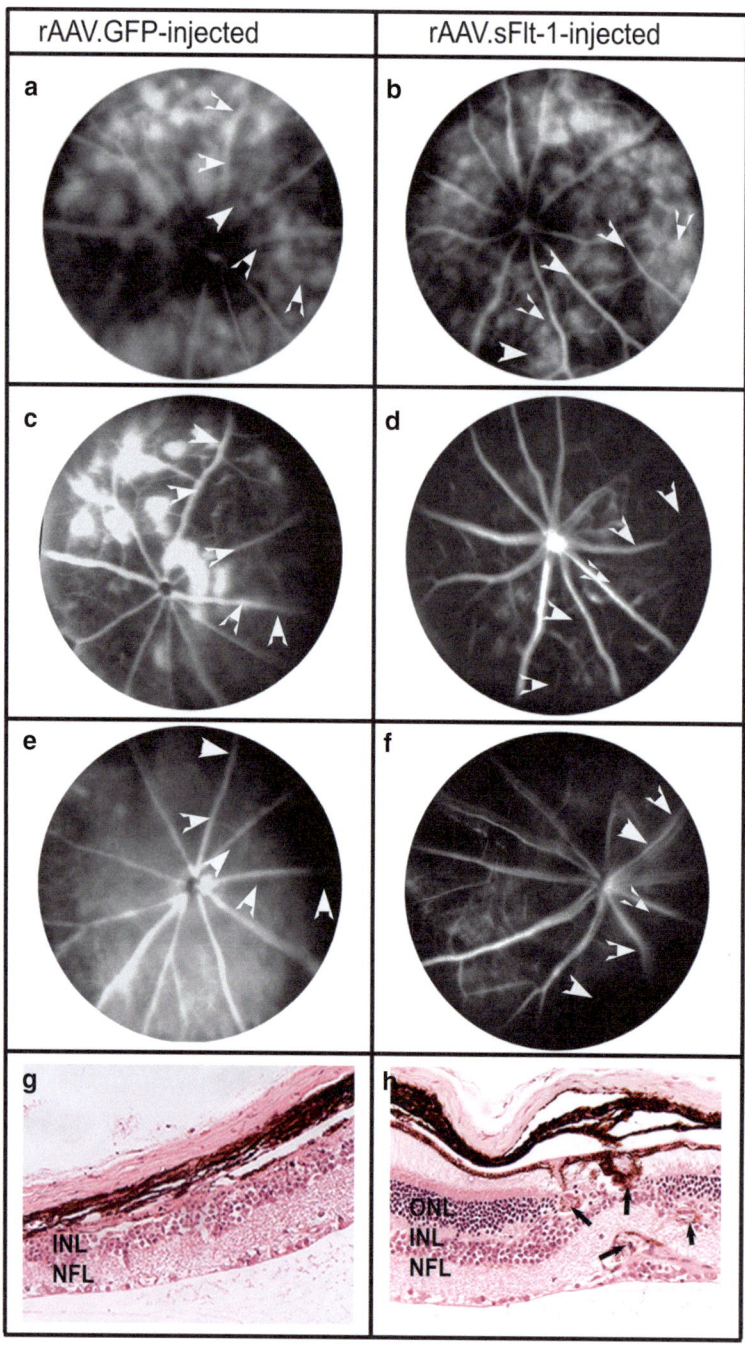

Histological analysis of the monkey eyes revealed no damage to the neural retinal cells, and no inflammatory response was observed in the non-lasered region of the macula at sites directly in contact with the injected rAAV vectors. In addition, sFlt-1 mRNA expression was detected in all monkey eyes injected with rAAV. sFlt-1 at 17 months after injection of the vector.

The findings in this monkey study suggested that there was long-term expression and activity of sFlt-1 17 months following subretinal injection. Importantly, subretinal administration of the vector was well tolerated and not associated with any toxicity (Lai et al. 2005b).

In a follow-up study conducted to assess whether the delivery of rAAV.sFlt-1 or sFlt-1 protein into the subretinal space of monkeys would affect retinal function, whether the vector (rAAV2) or the transgene product (sFlt-1) would elicit an immune response (immunogenicity studies), and also to assess whether the rAAV.sFlt-1 would be disseminated systemically (biodistribution studies), nine monkeys were used. One eye each of five monkeys was injected with rAAV.sFlt-1 in 100 μL of phosphate-buffered saline. One monkey was injected in both eyes, each with 10 μg of recombinant sFlt-1 protein in 100 μL of phosphate-buffered saline. Three monkeys were included as controls. One control monkey was kept as an uninjected control, and one eye each of two controls received rAAV.GFP (Lai et al. 2012). The retinal function of the monkeys was assessed by electroretinography (ERG). Amplitudes and implicit times from the responses of the injected eye and uninjected contralateral eye were calculated and compared preinjection and at different times following injection. There was no difference in any of the ERG measurements of retinal function between the treated and untreated eyes.

In the immunogenicity studies, immune response at different times following subretinal injection of rAAV.sFlt-1 was analyzed using a panel of antibodies that would identify changes in immune cell subset populations. No statistically significant changes in immune cell subset populations were observed. Additionally, a more in-depth study of circulating cells was conducted to assess the possibility that either the vector (rAAV) or the inserted gene product (sFlt-1) may cause immune activation. Using a small subset of phenotypic markers (HLA-DR, Ki-67, and Bcl-2), any signs of activation of CD4 or CD8 T cells and/or B cells following administration of rAAV.sFlt-1 were investigated. The data indicated that although there was a transient prolifera-

tive response in CD4 T cells, CD8 T cells, and B cells, this occurred independently of rAAV-sFlt-1 therapy, and the cells that proliferated did not display a standard activated effector phenotype. Altogether, these data suggested that rAAV.sFlt-1 therapy did not result in systemic immune activation (Lai et al. 2012). The overall positive findings and lack of toxicity of rAAV vectors in preclinical studies, as well as the findings with rAAV.sFlt-1 in mammalian models of CNV/ARMD, provided extensive supporting data that the vector had a favorable safety profile.

6.3 The Approval Process

By 2006, we had pharmacology results with rAAV.sFlt-1 injection in transgenic Kimba mice (Lai et al. 2005b), rats (Lai et al. 2002) and monkeys (Lai et al. 2005b). While completing the remaining preclinical studies, we began discussions with the regulatory agency to conduct a human trial with rAAV.sFlt-1. In 2006, no information was available on the use of gene therapy products in the human eye, and the Australian government set up the Gene and Related Therapies Research Advisory Panel (GTRAP) under the umbrella of the National Health and Medical Research Council to advise on gene therapy-related issues. Following a preliminary submission, we had an initial hearing in 2006. We requested that the trial be considered under the Clinical Trial Notification (CTN) Scheme – Notification of Intent to Supply Unapproved Therapeutic Goods. Unfortunately, GTRAP recommended a full submission under the Clinical Trial Exemption (CTX) scheme, with more stringent requirements that are normally used for the introduction of new pharmaceuticals under the Pharmaceutical Benefits Scheme of Australia, and this required additional preparation and increased regulatory oversight. We began preparing a submission incorporating permits from the Institutional Biosafety Committee, the Office of the Gene Technology Regulator, and the Institutional Human Research

Fig. 6.5 Phase I/II clinical trial design flowchart

rAAV.sFlt-1 Phase I Dose escalation trial
10^{10} vg **rAAV.sFlt-1 (3 patients) + Ranibizumab only (1 patient)→** 2 months data collection
If no drug related complications then
10^{11} vg **rAAV.sFlt-1 (3 patients) + Ranibizumab only (1 patient)→** 2 months data collection
If no drug related complications then
Start Phase IIa (40 patients).

Ethics Committee and submitted our initial CTX application by the end of 2008. After several modifications, we finally received permission to conduct a "A phase I randomised single controlled, dose escalating trial to establish the base line safety and efficacy following a single subretinal injection of rAAV.sFlt-1 into the eyes of patients with exudative age-related macular degeneration (ARMD)" in 2011 (https://clinicaltrial.gov; NCT01494805).

6.3.1 Description of the Clinical Trial

We received permission to recruit 24 patients into the trial which was subsequently raised to 48 patients (Fig. 6.5).

The trial has a unique design as it provides the best available treatment for all participating patients. Due to the fact that sFlt-1 "production" following the injection of rAAV.sFlt-1 reaches peak levels 6–8 weeks postinjection, subjects in the gene therapy treatment groups also receive a Lucentis® injection at the baseline visit and at day 28 to protect their eye from the consequences of neovascularization during this initial period. Following these two mandatory injections, Lucentis® is given on an "as needed" basis, using prespecified, objective re-treatment criteria.

6.3.2 The Manufacturing

The rAAV.sFlt-1 vector was manufactured in the Joint Vector Laboratories (JVL) at the University of North Carolina (UNC). The JVL current good manufacturing practice facility has extensive

experience in the preparation of rAAV vectors for use in early-stage clinical trials. The rAAV.sFlt-1 vector was produced using a pAAV.CMV.sFlt-1 plasmid encoding the human sFlt-1 gene. The pAAV.CMV.sFlt-1 plasmid was prepared by the Lions Eye Institute (LEI) in Perth, Western Australia, and shipped to the JVL for production of clinical-grade rAAV.sFlt-1 vector.

The major steps in rAAV.sFlt-1 vector production were described in the Introduction section of this book; thus, no details are given here. The product was released based on several release assays designed to measure identity, potency, and purity of the gene therapy product.

In addition to the release assays, we conducted additional tests at Molecular Ophthalmology, Lions Eye Institute, The University of Western Australia. The goal of this additional testing was to provide supporting information on the safety and potency of the product following shipment and further assure the quality of the investigational product.

The purpose of these tests was to demonstrate that the lot of rAAV.sFlt-1 produced for use in the clinical trial was (1) biologically active via its ability to inhibit VEGF-induced proliferation of Human Umbilical Vein Endothelial Cells (HUVEC) and (2) caused no gross toxicity following injection of rAAV.sFlt-1 into the subretinal space of mice.

1. The biological activity and inhibitory effect of sFlt-1 were confirmed by the inhibition of VEGF-driven HUVEC growth when rAAV.sFlt-1-conditioned media were added to HUVEC cultured in the media containing VEGF. In the presence of conditioned media from HEK 293 cells transduced with rAAV.sFlt-1, HUVEC cells grew significantly slower than the controls.

2. Following subretinal injection into mouse eyes with clinical-grade rAAV.sFlt-1, human sFlt-1 protein was detected around 1,500.0 pg/mL. There was no difference between phosphate-buffered saline-injected eyes and those injected with the clinical-grade rAAV.sFlt-1 at 4 weeks postinjection as examined by Spectralis HRA + OCT, Heidelberg. On the basis of these experiments, we recommended the commencement of the human clinical trial.

6.3.3 Initiation of Human Trials

The first patient was recruited on 16 December 2011. She was a 74-year-old female suffering from wet-ARMD. As an elderly patient, she had several comorbidities, including mild lymphopenia, but was deemed suitable for trial enrollment. She had active subfoveal CNV in the study eye with visual acuity of 37 Early Treatment Diabetic Retinopathy Study (ETDRS) letters. She received rAAV.sFlt-1 via subretinal injection on 5th January 2012, at a dose of 10^{10} genomes administered in 100 μl volume following vitrectomy and detachment of the posterior vitreous. The delivery of AAV.sFlt-1 resulted in the formation of a bleb under the retina with clear boundaries. After 24 h, most of the air in the vitreous had absorbed, and only a small mark at the site of subretinal injection remained visible.

6.3.4 The Results

Serial ophthalmic examinations over 12 months revealed no superficial, anterior segment, or vitreous inflammatory signs in the subject. There was no evidence of loss of visual acuity, intraocular pressure elevation, retinal detachment, or significant intraocular or systemic inflammation in the patient as of the last study visit. The patient suffered from mild lymphopenia at baseline, and her condition remained unchanged during the study period. There were no significant changes in any laboratory tests when compared to the baseline. There was a small amount of rAAV.

sFlt-1 detected in the tear sample of the injected eye that cleared within 2 weeks. Visual acuity improved by 7 ETDRS letters, and central retinal thickness decreased and remained stable beyond 1 year. During the first 12 months, the patient did not require any re-treatments with Lucentis (ranibizumab) or any other anti-VEGF therapy (Fig. 6.6). Within a period of 6 months six patients were injected with rAAV.sFlt-1 with no evidence of rAAV-related complications but with improvement in vision that was maintained at 12 months postinjection.

6.4 Future Plans

In 2012 and 2013, 38 patients were enrolled in the trial. Patient follow-up and data monitoring are ongoing. Following data analysis, the results will be reported in the relevant scientific journals.

6.5 Personal Observations

As a young girl (EPR), I heard about the success of the first heart transplant by Dr Christian Barnard in 1967. I decided to study medical science with the hope that, instead of helping tens of thousands as a doctor, by discovering new therapies, I could treat millions. The rAAV.sFlt-1 gene therapy project is the result of a 20-year long intense research program with rewards as well as tribulations. On a personal level, reaching the clinical trial phase has also been a dream come true. Working in medical science at a time when new concepts were taking root and making my own contribution to the field of gene therapy have been a fantastic journey. I have been lucky to work with a large number of highly committed students, basic and clinical scientists, and ophthalmologists without whom this project could have never been completed. I would like to thank my mentor and colleague Professor Ian Constable for his continuous support of my work and my deputy Dr May Lai for her invaluable contribution to this work. I also would like to acknowledge

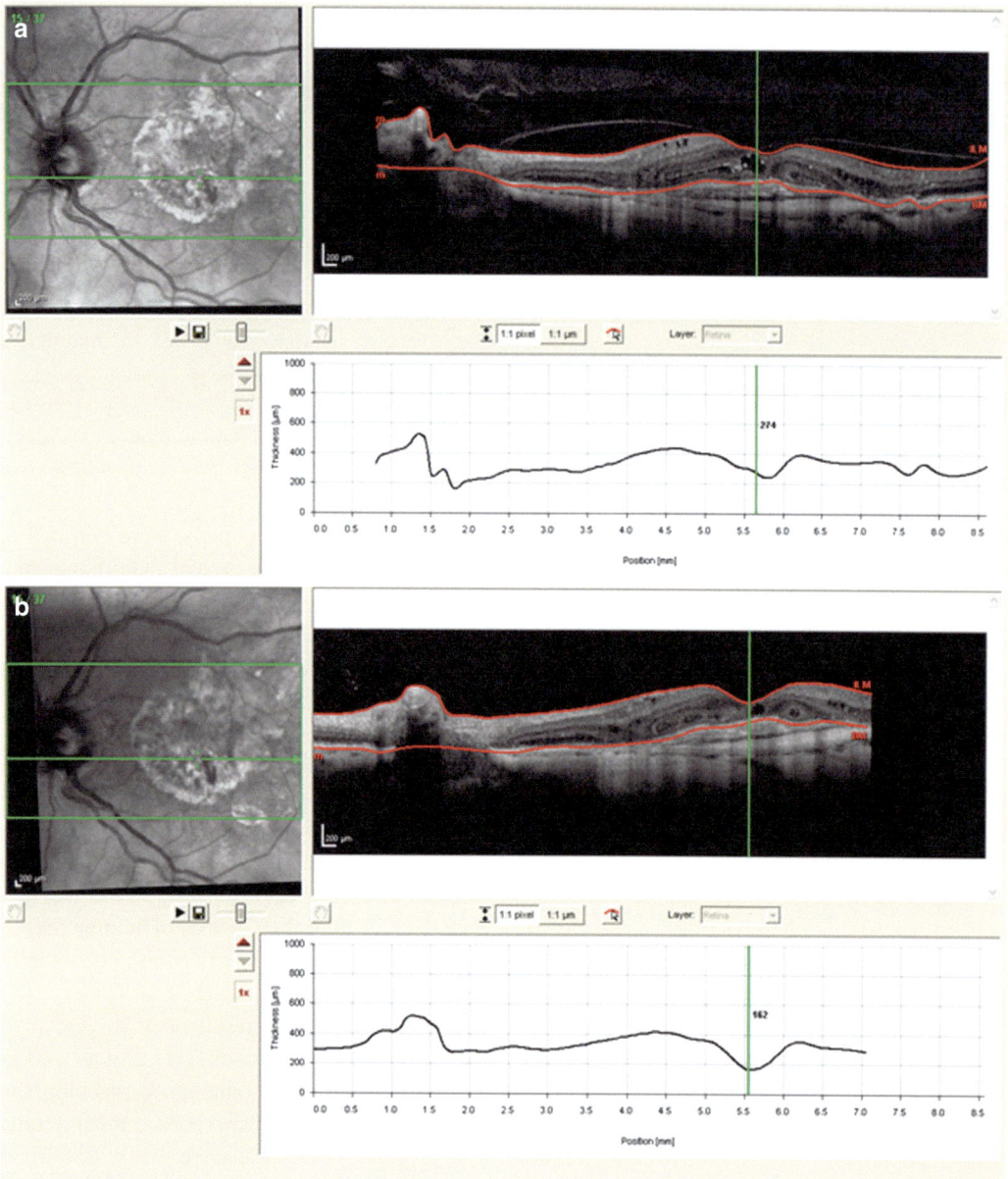

Fig. 6.6 Fluorescein angiography and optical coherence tomography (OCT) images of the patient's treated eye at baseline (**a**) and at 1 year (**b**) postinjection with rAAV.sFlt-1

the major funding agencies, the National Health and Medical Research Council of Australia and the Juvenile Diabetes Research Foundation, USA, that made the basic research phase possible and Avalanche Biotechnologies, Inc. for their support of the clinical trial phase.

During this journey, I have learned a lot about drug development and the regulatory process. We faced a significant challenge working on non-human primates, which were set up at the Singapore Eye Research Institute in Singapore. The GTRAP hearing and CTX application process were a significant undertaking and provided a unique opportunity for a small academic lab to navigate this challenging process.

Time will tell whether our approach will offer a safe and effective treatment for patients whose only current option involves frequent intravitreal injections. This therapy may also offer a cost-effective alternative to the expense and burden of currently available therapies. I am optimistic that we are at the dawn of a new era of vector-based biologics in ophthalmology, and it has been my extreme privilege to be part of the development of this field.

Compliance with Ethical Requirements Professors Elizabeth Rakoczy and Ian Constable provide consultancy for Avalanche Biotechnologies, Inc.

All procedures followed were in accordance with the ethical standards of the responsible committee on human experimentation (institutional and national) and with the Helsinki Declaration of 1975, as revised in 2000. Informed consent was obtained from all patients for being included in the study.

All institutional and national guidelines for the care and use of laboratory animals were followed. All experiments were approved by The University of Western Australia.

References

Acland GM, Aguirre GD, Ray J, Zhang Q, Aleman TS, Cideciyan AV, Pearce-Kelling SE, Anand V, Zeng Y, Maguire AM, Jacobson SG, Hauswirth WW, Bennett J (2001) Gene therapy restores vision in a canine model of childhood blindness. Nat Genet 28(1):92–95. doi:10.1038/Ng0501-92

Adamis AP, Miller JW, Bernal MT, D'Amico DJ, Folkman J, Yeo TK, Yeo KT (1994) Increased vascular endothelial growth factor levels in the vitreous of eyes with proliferative diabetic retinopathy. Am J Ophthalmol 118(4):445–450

Ali Rahman IS, Li CR, Lai CM, Rakoczy EP (2011) In vivo monitoring of VEGF-induced retinal damage in the Kimba mouse model of retinal neovascularization. Curr Eye Res 36(7):654–662. doi:10.3109/02713683.2010.551172

Amano S, Rohan R, Kuroki M, Tolentino M, Adamis AP (1998) Requirement for vascular endothelial growth factor in wound- and inflammation-related corneal neovascularization. Invest Ophthalmol Vis Sci 39(1):18–22

Auricchio A, Kobinger G, Anand V, Hildinger M, O'Connor E, Maguire AM, Wilson JM, Bennett J (2001) Exchange of surface proteins impacts on viral vector cellular specificity and transduction characteristics: the retina as a model. Hum Mol Genet 10(26):3075–3081

Barleon B, Totzke F, Herzog C, Blanke S, Kremmer E, Siemeister G, Marme D, Martiny-Baron G (1997) Mapping of the sites for ligand binding and receptor dimerization at the extracellular domain of the vascular endothelial growth factor receptor FLT-1. J Biol Chem 272(16):10382–10388

Bennett J, Maguire AM, Cideciyan AV, Schnell M, Glover E, Anand V, Aleman TS, Chirmule N, Gupta AR, Huang Y, Gao GP, Nyberg WC, Tazelaar J, Hughes J, Wilson JM, Jacobson SG (1999) Stable transgene expression in rod photoreceptors after recombinant adeno-associated virus-mediated gene transfer to monkey retina. Proc Natl Acad Sci U S A 96(17):9920–9925

Binz N, Ali Rahman IS, Chinnery HR, McKeone R, Simpson KM, Speed TP, Lai CM, Rakoczy PE (2013) Effect of vascular endothelial growth factor upregulation on retinal gene expression in the Kimba mouse. Clin Experiment Ophthalmol 41(3):251–262. doi:10.1111/j.1442-9071.2012.02845.x

Churchill AJ, Carter JG, Lovell HC, Ramsden C, Turner SJ, Yeung A, Escardo J, Atan D (2006) VEGF polymorphisms are associated with neovascular age-related macular degeneration. Hum Mol Genet 15(19):2955–2961. doi:10.1093/hmg/ddl238

de Vries C, Escobedo JA, Ueno H, Houck K, Ferrara N, Williams LT (1992) The fms-like tyrosine kinase, a receptor for vascular endothelial growth factor. Science 255(5047):989–991

Ferrara N (2004) Vascular endothelial growth factor: basic science and clinical progress. Endocr Rev 25(4):581–611. doi:10.1210/er.2003-0027

Folkman J, Merler E, Abernathy C, Williams G (1971) Isolation of a tumor factor responsible for angiogenesis. J Exp Med 133(2):275–288

Goldman CK, Kendall RL, Cabrera G, Soroceanu L, Heike Y, Gillespie GY, Siegal GP, Mao X, Bett AJ, Huckle WR, Thomas KA, Curiel DT (1998) Paracrine expression of a native soluble vascular endothelial growth factor receptor inhibits tumor growth, metastasis, and mortality rate. Proc Natl Acad Sci U S A 95(15):8795–8800

Kendall RL, Thomas KA (1993) Inhibition of vascular endothelial cell growth factor activity by an endogenously encoded soluble receptor. Proc Natl Acad Sci U S A 90(22):10705–10709

Kendall RL, Wang G, Thomas KA (1996) Identification of a natural soluble form of the vascular endothelial growth factor receptor, FLT-1, and its heterodimerization with KDR. Biochem Biophys Res Commun 226(2):324–328. doi:10.1006/bbrc.1996.1355

Kong HL, Hecht D, Song W, Kovesdi I, Hackett NR, Yayon A, Crystal RG (1998) Regional suppression of tumor growth by in vivo transfer of a cDNA encoding a secreted form of the extracellular domain of the flt-1 vascular endothelial growth factor receptor. Hum Gene Ther 9(6):823–833. doi:10.1089/hum.1998.9.6-823

Lai CM, Brankov M, Zaknich T, Lai YKY, Shen WY, Constable IJ, Kovesdi I, Rakoczy PE (2001)

Inhibition of angiogenesis by adenovirus-mediated sFlt-1 expression in a rat model of corneal neovascularization. Hum Gene Ther 12(10):1299–1310. doi:10.1089/104303401750270959

Lai YK, Shen WY, Brankov M, Lai CM, Constable IJ, Rakoczy PE (2002) Potential long-term inhibition of ocular neovascularisation by recombinant adeno-associated virus-mediated secretion gene therapy. Gene Ther 9(12):804–813. doi:10.1038/sj.gt.3301695

Lai CM, Dunlop SA, May LA, Gorbatov M, Brankov M, Shen WY, Binz N, Lai YK, Graham CE, Barry CJ, Constable IJ, Beazley LD, Rakoczy EP (2005a) Generation of transgenic mice with mild and severe retinal neovascularisation. Br J Ophthalmol 89(7):911–916. doi:10.1136/bjo.2004.059089

Lai CM, Shen WY, Brankov M, Lai YK, Barnett NL, Lee SY, Yeo IY, Mathur R, Ho JE, Pineda P, Barathi A, Ang CL, Constable IJ, Rakoczy EP (2005b) Long-term evaluation of AAV-mediated sFlt-1 gene therapy for ocular neovascularization in mice and monkeys. Mol Ther 12(4):659–668. doi:10.1016/j.ymthe.2005.04.022

Lai CM, Estcourt MJ, Wikstrom M, Himbeck RP, Barnett NL, Brankov M, Tee LB, Dunlop SA, Degli-Esposti MA, Rakoczy EP (2009) rAAV.sFlt-1 gene therapy achieves lasting reversal of retinal neovascularization in the absence of a strong immune response to the viral vector. Invest Ophthalmol Vis Sci 50(9):4279–4287. doi:10.1167/iovs.08-3253

Lai CM, Estcourt MJ, Himbeck RP, Lee SY, Yew-San Yeo I, Luu C, Loh BK, Lee MW, Barathi A, Villano J, Ang CL, van der Most RG, Constable IJ, Dismuke D, Samulski RJ, Degli-Esposti MA, Rakoczy EP (2012) Preclinical safety evaluation of subretinal AAV2.sFlt-1 in non-human primates. Gene Ther 19(10):999–1009. doi:10.1038/gt.2011.169

Leung DW, Cachianes G, Kuang WJ, Goeddel DV, Ferrara N (1989) Vascular endothelial growth factor is a secreted angiogenic mitogen. Science 246(4935):1306–1309

Narfstrom K, Bragadottir R, Redmond TM, Rakoczy PE, van Veen T, Bruun A (2003a) Functional and structural evaluation after AAV.RPE65 gene transfer in the canine model of Leber's congenital amaurosis. Adv Exp Med Biol 533:423–430

Narfstrom K, Katz ML, Bragadottir R, Seeliger M, Boulanger A, Redmond TM, Caro L, Lai CM, Rakoczy PE (2003b) Functional and structural recovery of the retina after gene therapy in the RPE65 null mutation dog. Invest Ophthalmol Vis Sci 44(4):1663–1672

Narfstrom K, Seeliger M, Lai CM, Vaegan, Katz M, Rakoczy EP, Reme C (2008) Morphological aspects related to long-term functional improvement of the retina in the 4 years following rAAV-mediated gene transfer in the RPE65 null mutation dog. Adv Exp Med Biol 613:139–146

Rakoczy EP, Ali Rahman IS, Binz N, Li CR, Vagaja NN, de Pinho M, Lai CM (2010) Characterization of a mouse model of hyperglycemia and retinal neovascularization. Am J Pathol 177(5):2659–2670. doi:10.2353/ajpath.2010.090883

Rolling F, Shen WY, Tabarias H, Constable I, Kanagasingam Y, Barry CJ, Rakoczy PE (1999) Evaluation of adeno-associated virus-mediated gene transfer into the rat retina by clinical fluorescence photography. Hum Gene Ther 10(4):641–648. doi:10.1089/10430349950018715

Rolling F, Shen WY, Barnett NL, Tabarias H, Kanagasingam Y, Constable I, Rakoczy PE (2000) Long-term real-time monitoring of adeno-associated virus-mediated gene expression in the rat retina. Clin Experiment Ophthalmol 28(5):382–386. doi:10.1046/j.1442-9071.2000.00341.x

Samulski RJ, Chang LS, Shenk T (1989) Helper-free stocks of recombinant adeno-associated viruses: normal integration does not require viral gene expression. J Virol 63(9):3822–3828

Sandercoe TM, Geller SF, Hendrickson AE, Stone J, Provis JM (2003) VEGF expression by ganglion cells in central retina before formation of the foveal depression in monkey retina: evidence of developmental hypoxia. J Comp Neurol 462(1):42–54. doi:10.1002/cne.10705

Shen WY, Lee SY, Yeo IYS, Lai C-M, Mathur R, Tan D, Constable IJ, Rakoczy PE (2004) Predilection of the macular region to high incidence of choroidal neovascularization after intense laser photocoagulation in the monkey. Arch Ophthalmol 122:353–360

Shen WY, Yu MJ, Barry CJ, Constable IJ, Rakoczy PE (1998) Expression of cell adhesion molecules and vascular endothelial growth factor in experimental choroidal neovascularisation in the rat. Br J Ophthalmol 82(9):1063–1071

Tee LB, Penrose MA, O'Shea JE, Lai CM, Rakoczy EP, Dunlop SA (2008) VEGF-induced choroidal damage in a murine model of retinal neovascularisation. Br J Ophthalmol 92(6):832–838. doi:10.1136/bjo.2007.130898

Trujillo CA, Nery AA, Alves JM, Martins AH, Ulrich H (2007) Development of the anti-VEGF aptamer to a therapeutic agent for clinical ophthalmology. Clin Ophthalmol 1(4):393–402

Vagaja NN, Chinnery HR, Binz N, Kezic JM, Rakoczy EP, McMenamin PG (2012) Changes in murine hyalocytes are valuable early indicators of ocular disease. Invest Ophthalmol Vis Sci 53(3):1445–1451. doi:10.1167/iovs.11-8601

Wulff C, Wilson H, Rudge JS, Wiegand SJ, Lunn SF, Fraser HM (2001) Luteal angiogenesis: prevention and intervention by treatment with vascular endothelial growth factor trap(A40). J Clin Endocrinol Metab 86(7):3377–3386

Transplantation of Human Embryonic Stem Cell-Derived Retinal Pigment Epithelium for the Treatment of Macular Degeneration

7

Aaron Nagiel, Robert Lanza, and Steven D. Schwartz

7.1 Introduction

The pathogenesis and treatment of age-related macular degeneration (AMD) are detailed in Chap. 5. Below we describe the most common form of juvenile-onset macular degeneration known as Stargardt's macular dystrophy. In addition, a brief primer on the science and history of retinal pigment epithelium (RPE) transplantation for these conditions is provided.

7.1.1 Hereditary Macular Dystrophies

Despite their rarity, there has been substantial interest in the classification and treatment of hereditary macular dystrophies. Over 100 specific genetic loci have been identified for retinal

A. Nagiel, MD, PhD
Jules Stein Eye Institute, David Geffen School of Medicine, University of California, Los Angeles, Los Angeles, CA, USA

Department of Ophthalmology, University of California, Los Angeles, Los Angeles, CA, USA

R. Lanza
Advanced Cell Technology, Marlborough, MA, USA

S.D. Schwartz (✉)
Retina Division, Jules Stein Eye Institute, David Geffen School of Medicine, University of California, Los Angeles, Los Angeles, CA, USA
e-mail: schwartz@jsei.ucla.edu

dystrophies (Koenekoop et al. 2007), and this creates enormous potential for understanding the pathogenesis of retinal degenerations and makes it conceivable to replace the specific genes or cell types affected by the disorder. Many of the genes implicated in macular dystrophies are expressed by the RPE and lead to RPE dysfunction and eventual apoptosis when mutated.

The most common juvenile-onset macular degeneration is Stargardt's macular dystrophy with an estimated prevalence of 1 in 10,000–15,000 individuals (Travis et al. 2007). It initially presents in the first or second decade with decreased visual acuity and classic examination findings such as retinal flecks, a central atrophic maculopathy, and relative hypofluorescence of the choroid on fluorescein angiography ("dark choroid" sign). Many patients progress to geographic atrophy that affects the central vision. This phenotype has been linked to several genes, but the most common form is an autosomal recessive mutation in the *ABCA4* transporter gene (Koenekoop 2003; Sun and Nathans 1997). The defective transporter protein impairs clearance of all-trans-retinaldehyde from photoreceptor outer segments and leads to accumulation of toxic lipofuscin fluorophores in the RPE (Weng et al. 1999).

In order to directly address the genetic defect in Stargardt's patients, there is currently one Phase I/IIa clinical trial underway in humans utilizing lentiviral vector delivery of the *ABCA4* gene (clinical trial NCT01367444). This is a promising therapeutic approach for this disease and for other maculopathies with a known genetic basis. One limitation to gene-based therapies, however, is that they are unlikely to provide a benefit in moderate to advanced cases where RPE loss has already occurred. Another treatment approach would be to replace the diseased or missing RPE with healthy RPE cells that can sustainably integrate into the compromised RPE monolayer. This approach may be successful even in diseases such as Stargardt's where the defective protein is expressed in photoreceptors but leads to deleterious effects on the RPE. Transplanting healthy RPE in such cases might treat the disease by temporarily stalling the atrophic process and visual loss—and could be used as a supplement to gene-replacement therapy.

7.1.2 Cell-Based Therapies for Macular Degeneration

The transplantation of undifferentiated or differentiated cells into specific anatomical locations for therapeutic effect holds great promise, especially for the treatment of retinal disease (Pan et al. 2013). Although gene-delivery approaches are advantageous in that they directly replace the missing or dysfunctional protein, the major drawback is that the creation of individual delivery vectors is tedious and the therapy is of unclear benefit when the target cells have already been lost to disease. Cell replacement is advantageous in that it can be applied to any disease process with the common endpoint being damage to a specific cell type.

The retina is an especially promising site for the delivery of cell-based therapies. First, we can deliver the cells and observe their effect under direct visualization using ophthalmoscopy and with high-resolution optical coherence tomography (OCT). Second, the subretinal space is an immune-privileged site with markedly diminished cellular and humoral responses (Wenkel and Streilein 1998), which may limit the rejection of foreign cells. Third, the laminar architecture of the retina allows for cells to be delivered to a specific location without requiring the cells

to migrate. RPE cell transplantation is particularly advantageous in that these cells do not require synapse formation once targeted to the subretinal space. Fourth, a successful therapeutic effect can be quantified using many functional measures including visual acuity, visual field testing, microperimetry, color vision, contrast sensitivity, and dark adaptation.

RPE cell transplants have been tested in animal models of macular degeneration for almost 30 years. The initial studies were facilitated by the successful in vitro culture and characterization of adult human RPE cells (Flood et al. 1980). A few years later, the same group was able to transplant these cultured cells into monkey eyes (Gouras et al. 1984, 1985). The first report of a therapeutic benefit to RPE transplantation came when Lopez et al. successfully transplanted dissociated RPE cells from normal rats into the Royal College of Surgeons (RCS) rats (Lopez et al. 1989), which suffer from a panretinal degeneration due to a defect in photoreceptor phagocytosis (Gal et al. 2000). The transplanted RPE cells were shown to integrate in the host RPE layer and phagocytose copious amounts of photoreceptor outer segment material. The first attempt at RPE transplantation in humans reported the placement of an RPE flap or allogeneic RPE cells in two eyes with advanced AMD in which subretinal fibrosis had occurred (Peyman et al. 1991). A concern with such approaches in humans has been the risk of transplant rejection. One solution to this problem would be to use autologous RPE cells or grafts from the host eye and transplanting them into diseased areas (Binder et al. 2002). However, this approach has been fraught with difficulties including insufficient tissue material, clumping of the transplanted RPE (Del Priore et al. 2001), proliferative vitreoretinopathy at the site of harvesting (van Meurs et al. 2004), and whether autologous cells will be susceptible to the same disease process.

Human embryonic stem cells stand as an attractive and potentially unlimited source of RPE for use in transplantation. Klimanskaya et al. were the first to successfully differentiate hESCs into RPE and then inject these cells into the RCS rat model (Klimanskaya et al. 2004;

Lu et al. 2009; Lund et al. 2006). Remarkably, the transplanted cells preserved the photoreceptor layer even when as few as 20,000 cells were injected. A similar result was found when these cells were injected into ELOVL4 mutant mice, a mouse model for Stargardt's macular dystrophy. Besides the risk of graft rejection, a major concern with these studies is the possibility of teratoma or tumor formation as has been reported upon injection of less differentiated hESC precursors (Arnhold et al. 2004). However, preclinical studies in animals that utilized differentiated RPE did not find any evidence of abnormal cell proliferation (Lu et al. 2009; Lund et al. 2007).

The long history of RPE transplantation for macular disease has been fraught with difficulty, but work on animal models using human embryonic stem cell-derived RPE (hESC-RPE) was very encouraging. In collaboration with Dr. Robert Lanza and his team at Advanced Cell Technologies, we embarked on the first human clinical trial exploring the use of hESC-RPE in the treatment with dry AMD and Stargardt's macular dystrophy (clinical trials NCT01345006 and NCT01344993).

7.2   The Road to Stem Cell-Derived RPE Transplants in Humans

In order to perform the first stem cell-derived RPE transplants in humans, we undertook a long and arduous journey of over 10 years. Like all basic science research, the preclinical in vitro and animal work was riddled with failures and disappointments. However, with the persistence and dedication of Dr. Lanza and his team, we were able to successfully create hESC-RPE suitable for use in human clinical trials. Ironically, the most difficult time for us was not the scientific development phase but rather obtaining regulatory and institutional approval. The Federal Drug Administration (FDA) approval process was appropriately rigorous, but our interactions were cordial, positive, and educational. Realizing that close scrutiny of this study was appropriate given the groundbreaking nature of the work, the

University Institutional Review Board and Bioethics approvals were in some ways more challenging than obtaining an investigational new drug (IND) number from the FDA. Thankfully, the University of California at Los Angeles research infrastructure has been down this road before, and recognizing the potential impact of the work, we were given the green light to proceed with our clinical trials.

7.3   Deriving RPE from Human Embryonic Stem Cells

The prospect of using RPE differentiated from hESCs for transplantation in humans posed several key advantages. A potentially unlimited supply of differentiated young cells could be created in vitro and extensively tested for differentiation markers, pathogens, functional assays, and genotype to ensure the quality of the cells. In addition, hESCs and their differentiated progeny have been shown in several studies to exhibit decreased immunogenicity, perhaps diminishing the possibility of rejection after transplantation (Drukker et al. 2006; Okamura et al. 2007).

With the eventual goal of using these cells in humans, it was imperative that we generate pure, pathogen-free, and differentiated RPE cells. In our initial preclinical work, we used the MA09 hESC cell line to create a master cell bank with Good Manufacturing Practices (Klimanskaya et al. 2004). These cells were expanded on mitomycin-C-treated mouse embryonic fibroblasts for three passages. Upon allowing the cells to differentiate in culture, we noted that many of the cells expressed a neuronal phenotype (PAX6 positive and TUBULIN β III positive). Over time, some of the epithelioid cells appeared as polygonal pigmented cells, and we were able to manually isolate these patches of putative RPE cells. Figure 7.1a illustrates the patches of RPE that formed in the differentiating culture of embryoid bodies. We trypsinized these cell clumps, purified them, and then subjected the cells to extensive testing, including pathogen, karyotyping, phagocytosis assays, differentiation and purity, quantitative PCR, and quantitative immunostaining for

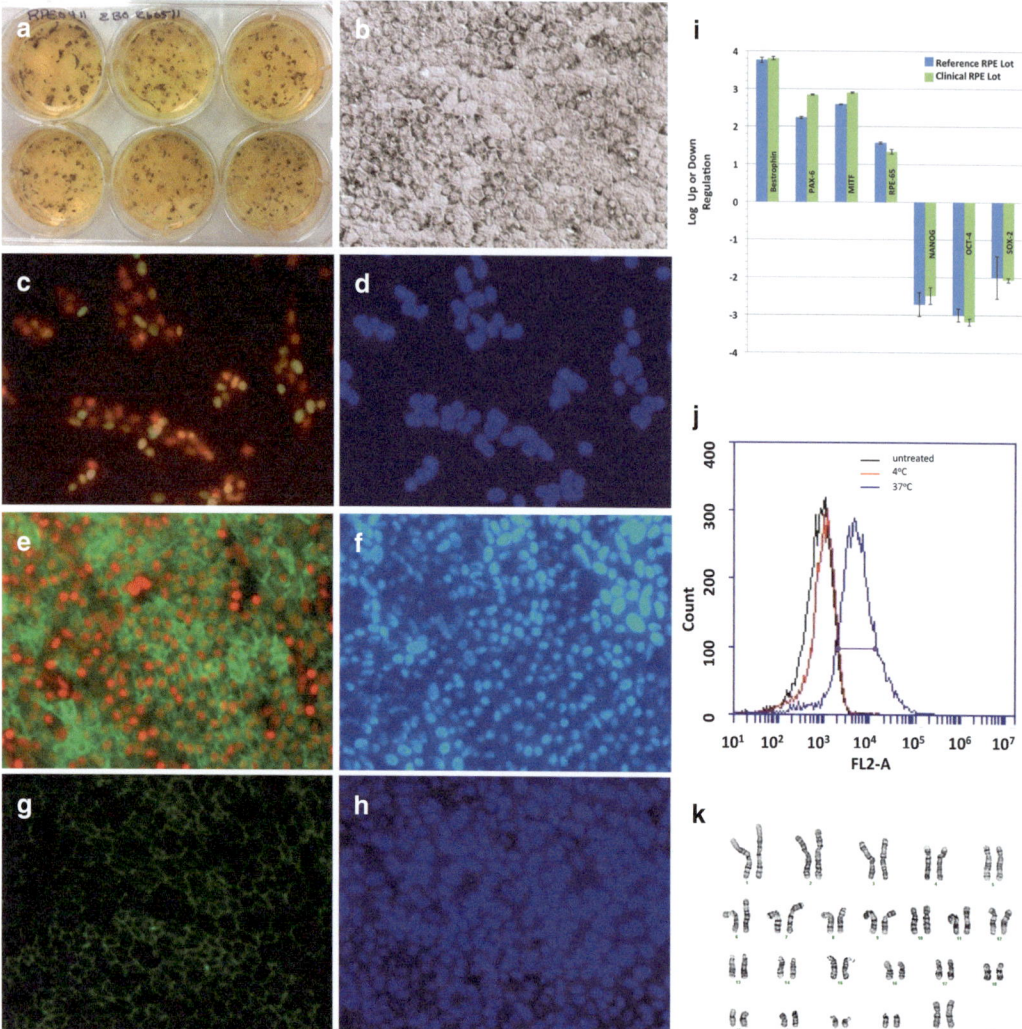

Fig. 7.1 Cellular and molecular characterization of RPE cells derived from human embryonic stem cells. (**a**) A six-well dish with pigmented RPE cell patches in the differentiating culture of embryoid bodies. (**b**) Photomicrograph of 3-week-old hESC-RPE showing a confluent monolayer of medium pigmented cells. (**c–d**) Immunofluorescence for MITF (*red*) and PAX6 (*green*) in (c) and the corresponding DAPI (*blue*) image in (d). (**e–f**) Immunofluorescence for bestrophin (*red*) and PAX6 (*green*) in (e) and the corresponding DAPI (*blue*) image in (f). (**g–h**) Immunofluorescence for ZO-1 (*green*) in (g) and the corresponding DAPI (*blue*) in (h). (**i**) Quantitative PCR for RPE and hESC markers performed on a reference RPE cell lot and the hESC-RPE cell lot. (**j**) Flow cytometry histogram showing phagocytosis of pH-sensitive fluorescent bioparticles at 37 and 4 °C. (**k**) Normal female karyotype (46 XX) of the hESC-RPE lot (Reprinted from Schwartz et al. (2012), Copyright (2012), with permission from Elsevier)

RPE and hESC markers. Microscopic analysis demonstrated the purified in vitro RPE cultures to have normal epithelial morphology with light to medium pigmentation and strongly expressed the differentiation markers PAX6 and MITF (Fig. 7.1b–f). Quantitative PCR for RPE and stem cell markers showed strong upregulation of the RPE markers bestrophin, PAX6, MITF, and RPE65 and downregulation of the hESC markers NANOG, OCT4, and SOX2. These values were identical to those found in a reference RPE set (Fig. 7.1i). The purified RPE cells displayed robust phagocytic activity as measured by their ingestion of pHrodo bioparticles at 37 °C

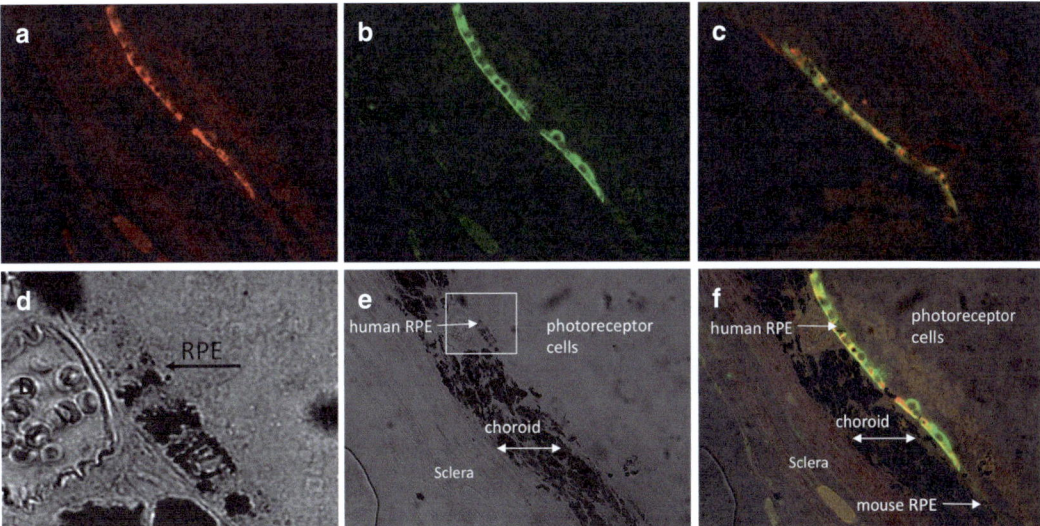

Fig. 7.2 Engraftment of hESC-RPE cells into NIH III immune-nude mice 9 months after subretinal injection. Mouse eye section stained with anti-human mitochondria (**a**) and anti-human bestrophin (**b**). Human mitochondria and bestrophin colocalize in the same cell (**c**). (**e**) Bright-field microscope image of the section in (a) and (b) with inset (**d**) showing structure of the engrafted hESC-RPE. (**f**) Merged image of (a, b, and e) showing hESC-RPE alongside host mouse RPE (Reprinted from Schwartz et al. (2012), Copyright (2012), with permission from Elsevier)

(Fig. 7.1j). In addition, the karyotype of the purified RPE cells was normal (Fig. 7.1k).

After demonstrating that our purified cells harbored normal RPE characteristics and were pathogen-free, we injected the cells into animal models for efficacy and safety analysis (Lu et al. 2009). hESC-RPE cells were injected subretinally in RCS and Elovl4 mutant mice. The transplanted cells successfully integrated into the RPE monolayer and survived there for more than 8 months without evidence of tumor formation. Strikingly, the transplanted cells endowed the mice with improved visual acuity and luminance threshold response. In addition, human RPE cells transplanted into NIH III immune-deficient mice remained localized to the subretinal space with no evidence of tumorigenicity, teratoma formation, or spread to other body parts (Fig. 7.2).

As a final step utilizing these cells in human subjects, we tested whether the degree of differentiation as measured by the melanin content per cell had an effect on the adhesion and growth of the cells. We harvested two separate lots of cells with different levels of pigmentation. After extrusion through the injection cannula, the cells were plated onto gelatin-coated wells and monitored for attachment and growth. The lighter pigmented lot had a much higher initial attachment rate with fewer floating cells (Fig. 7.3a–d). After 4 days in culture, the cell density was significantly higher for the lighter lot than the darker lot (Fig. 7.3e–g). We proceeded to use this lighter RPE lot for clinical testing in humans under the hypothesis that these cells would more easily survive the transplantation process and adhere to Bruch's membrane.

7.4   The First hESC-Derived RPE Transplants in Humans

Given the extensive in vitro testing and the promising results from preclinical animal models, we felt justified in proceeding to human trials. This effort would represent the first ever hESC-derived RPE transplantation in human beings. Our institution's Clinical Research Center aided us substantially in the preparation and planning for the trial. The trial would be a Phase I/Phase II safety and efficacy trial and at first enroll only two patients: one with dry AMD and one with Stargardt's macular dystrophy. We selected

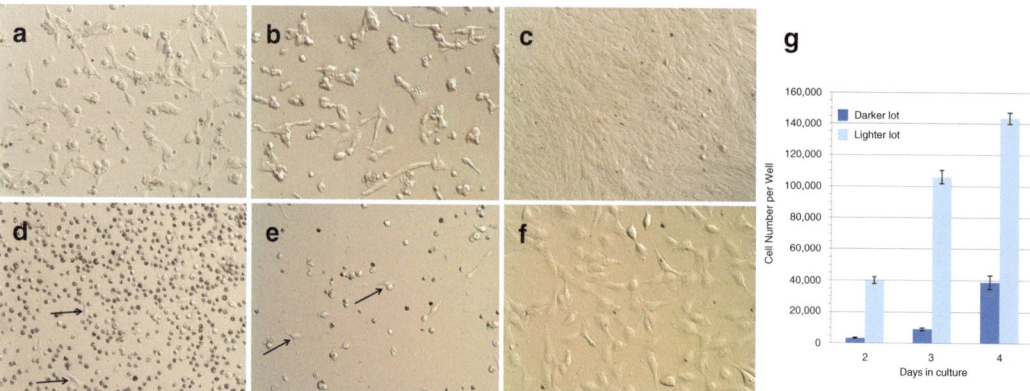

Fig. 7.3 Comparison of attachment and growth of hESC-RPE depending on degree of cell pigmentation. Micrographs of lightly pigmented cells (**a, c, e**) and darkly pigmented cells (**b, d, f**) plated onto gelatin-coated dishes. (**a, b**) Micrographs of cells 21 h after plating, with many cells in the pigmented lot (**b**) unattached. (**c, d**) The same cultures after removal of floating cells. *Arrows* in (**d**) show attached cells. (**e, f**) Cultures at 3 days after plating with the lighter cells (**e**) displaying greater cell numbers in a confluent monolayer. (**g**) Attachment and proliferation of lighter and darker hESC-RPE lots after plating (Reprinted from Schwartz et al. (2012), Copyright (2012), with permission from Elsevier)

patients using extensive inclusion and exclusion criteria, including end-stage disease, central visual loss, the absence of other ocular diseases, no history of cancer, no contraindications for systemic immunosuppression, the ability to undergo surgery, and psychological suitability to participate in this experimental trial. Both patients provided informed consent and ethical approval was obtained from the University of California, Los Angeles, institutional review board. Prior to undergoing treatment, the patients underwent extensive baseline imaging and testing, including visual acuity, contrast sensitivity, fluorescein angiography, spectral domain optical coherence tomography (SD-OCT), and Goldmann visual field testing. Based upon these studies, we carefully selected a transplantation site in the paracentral macula that appeared compromised but not completely atrophic based on SD-OCT imaging. We believed that transplantation to an area with advanced atrophy would provide little benefit and would not simulate future studies in which these transplants would take place in less advanced eyes.

On the day of the procedure, vials of cryopreserved hESC-RPE cells were thawed and reconstituted to a density of 333 RPE cells per μl. With a planned injection volume of 150 μl, this would deliver the target dose of 50,000 viable RPE cells

into the subretinal space of each patient's eye. In the operating room, we performed a pars plana vitrectomy including surgical induction of a posterior vitreous detachment. The cells were injected through a small retinotomy using a 25-gauge MedOne PolyTip cannula directly into the submacular space near the preselected site of transplantation. Both vitrectomies were uneventful and the patients had an unremarkable postoperative course. The subretinal bleb flattened within 4 h of the procedure. There was no evidence of anterior segment inflammation or corneal edema in either patient. Fluorescein angiography and SD-OCT revealed no sign of inflammation, edema, or hyperproliferation up to 4 months after the transplantation. Both patients were started on an immunosuppressive regimen 1 week before surgery consisting of low-dose tacrolimus and mycophenolate mofetil, to be continued for 6 weeks. At this point, the regimen specifies a discontinuation of tacrolimus and continuing mycophenolate for an additional 6 weeks.

Although our utmost objective in this preliminary trial was to ensure the safety and feasibility of this transplantation paradigm, we were of course interested in anatomic and functional outcomes. We were unable to definitively identify any engrafted RPE in the AMD patient. Unfortunately, this patient had stopped taking the

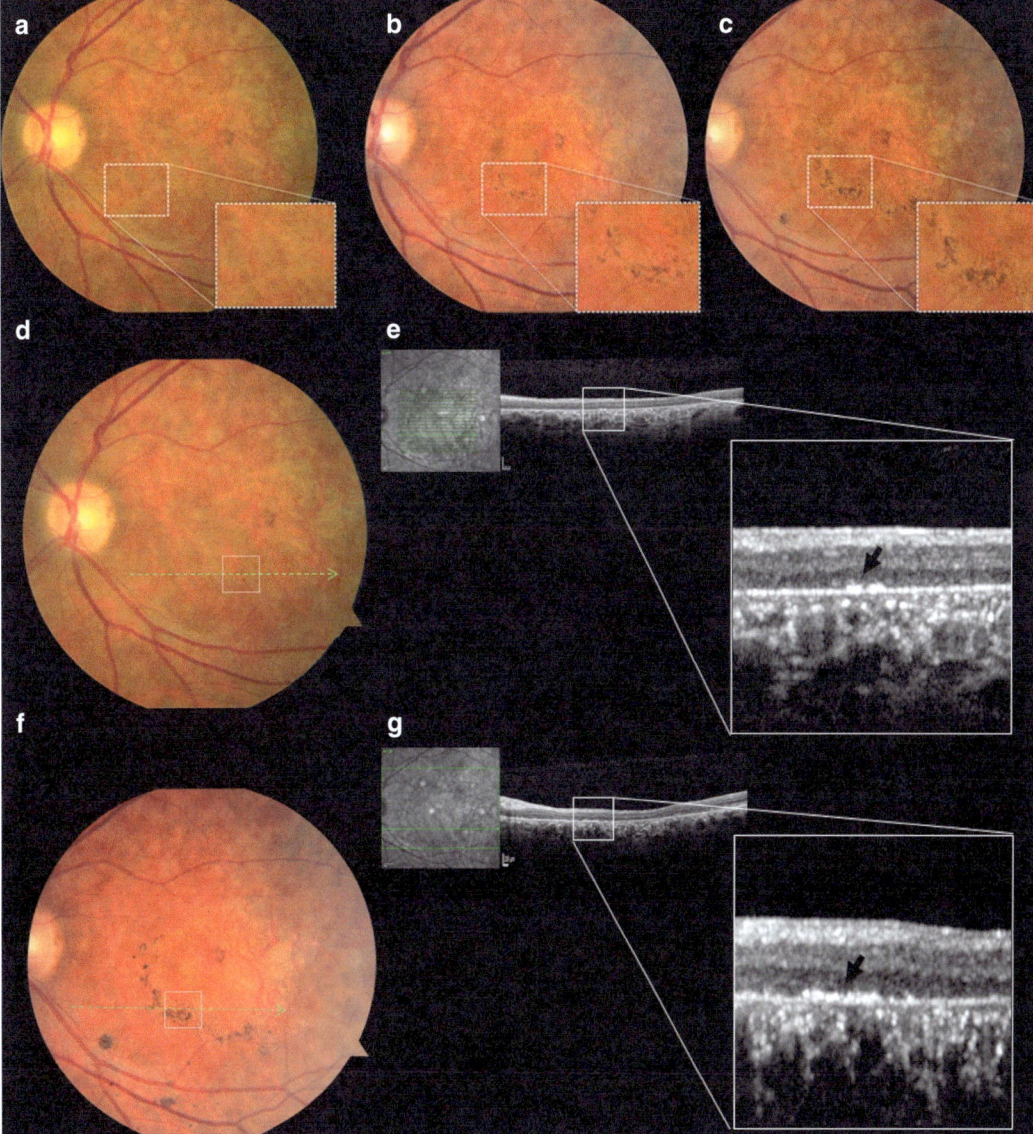

Fig. 7.4 Color fundus images and OCT of the hESC-RPE transplantation site in the patient with Stargardt's macular dystrophy. (**a**) Baseline color image shows extensive macular atrophy. (**b**) 1 week after transplantation, there is increased pigmentation in a region of atrophy at baseline. (**c**) At week 6 after transplantation, the pigmentation is even more evident. Baseline color fundus images (**d**) and OCT (**e**) showing widespread atrophy. (**f**, **g**) At month 3, there is increased pigmentation (**f**) which corresponds to increased reflectivity at the level of the RPE on OCT (*arrow*, **g**) (Reprinted from Schwartz et al. (2012), Copyright (2012), with permission from Elsevier)

immunosuppressive regimen during the first postoperative week. In the Stargardt's patient, we saw clear evidence of RPE engraftment. There was clinically evident pigmentation visible on biomicroscopy in the bed of the transplant, and these areas of increased pigmentation corresponded to areas of RPE engraftment on SD-OCT imaging (Fig. 7.4).

We next sought to identify functional outcomes resulting from successful RPE transplantation. Although the AMD patient did not show clinical evidence of engraftment and had stopped taking the

Table 7.1 Postoperative visual acuity in patient with Stargardt's macular dystrophy

	Fellow eye		Operated eye	
	BCVA	ETDRS letters	BCVA	ETDRS letters
Baseline	HM	0	HM	0
1 week	HM	0	CF	0
2 weeks	HM	0	CF	1
3 weeks	HM	0	CF	3
4 weeks	HM	0	20/800	5
6 weeks	HM	0	20/800	5
8 weeks	HM	0	20/800	5
12 weeks	HM	0	20/800	5

immunosuppressants, her Early Treatment of Diabetic Retinopathy Study (ETDRS) visual acuity improved slightly postoperatively from 20/500 to 20/320 at postoperative month 3. Goldmann visual field testing showed no visual field loss after the surgery and suggested a slight improvement. During this time period, the patient's untreated fellow eye also demonstrated mild improvements, making the outcomes in the treated eye difficult to interpret. In contrast, the patient with Stargardt's macular dystrophy had definite improvements in visual function (Table 7.1). The visual acuity preoperatively was hand motions and improved to count fingers by 2 weeks and then 20/800 by 3 months postoperatively. The Goldmann visual field was stable or slightly improved after the surgery. Of note, the fellow eye demonstrated no visual improvement.

We have been extremely encouraged by the results of this preliminary clinical trial utilizing hESC-RPE in two forms of macular degeneration. The Stargardt's patient showed clear evidence of engraftment of the transplanted RPE with a corresponding improvement in visual acuity. Although the AMD patient had no clear improvement in visual function, the most important result of this study is that neither patient was harmed by the intervention. Both patients had an uneventful postoperative course with no evidence of inflammation, excess cell proliferation, teratoma formation, or rejection of the transplanted cells. The persistent attachment of the transplanted RPE to Bruch's is very encouraging, but it remains unclear whether these cells will eventually succumb to disease or undergo rejection in the long term.

7.5 Future Plans

Our experience with these two patients excited us immensely about the prospect of completing the ongoing clinical trials and expanding the scope of this work. We were quite convinced that the Stargardt's patient had subjectively improved visual function. Most importantly, neither patient experienced an adverse event such as teratoma formation, retinal detachment, inflammation, or apparent rejection. However, this pioneering trial will leave many questions unanswered, and it is these questions that provide a scaffold for what needs to be done in future work. The three major emphasis points for any subsequent clinical trial include: (1) enrolling more patients in order to provide statistical significance, (2) recruiting patients with less advanced disease and thus greater potential for visual and anatomic recovery, and (3) testing the possibility of withholding systemic immunosuppression as this could significant expand the safety profile of the treatment if it could be shown to be noninferior.

With these goals, and supplemented with safety data from a number of subsequent patients treated in both trials, we applied for and received regulatory approval to expand the scope of the dry AMD and Stargardt's trials—work that is currently underway. First, we have assembled a multicenter collaborative effort with 5 academic centers (UCLA, Massachusetts Eye and Ear Infirmary, Wills Eye Institute, Bascom Palmer Eye Institute, and Moorfields). Second, patients with less advanced disease are being included with the goal of testing the hypothesis that earlier intervention may allow for better outcomes. Third, a portion of the patients included in subsequent trials will likely not be treated with systemic immunosuppressants in order to determine if they are truly necessary to prevent rejection.

Much rests on the outcome of these ongoing and future trials. The road to proving safety and efficacy is long with any new agent, but particularly so with complex biologic therapeutics like human embryonic stem cell-derived RPE for transplantation into the submacular space. Given the large numbers of patients with the target conditions, the unmet medical need, and the profound impact blindness has on the individual and on society, the enormity of the research efforts seems dwarfed by the potential to reduce common, untreatable blindness. It is our hope that these preliminary publications serve to promote successful stem cell research by sharing our detailed methods and by motivating funding bodies to support research utilizing complex biologic therapeutics.

Compliance with Ethical Requirements Aaron Nagiel and Steven D. Schwartz declare that they have no conflict of interest. Robert Lanza is an employee of Advanced Cell Technology, a biotechnology company in the area of stem cells and regenerative medicine.

All procedures followed were in accordance with the ethical standards of the responsible committee on human experimentation (institutional and national) and with the Helsinki Declaration of 1975, as revised in 2000. FDA, IRB, and ethics committee approval was secured prior to enrolling patients. Informed consent was obtained from all patients included in the study.

All institutional and national guidelines for the care and use of laboratory animals were followed.

References

Arnhold S, Klein H, Semkova I, Addicks K, Schraermeyer U (2004) Neurally selected embryonic stem cells induce tumor formation after long-term survival following engraftment into the subretinal space. Invest Ophthalmol Vis Sci 45:4251–4255

Binder S, Stolba U, Krebs I, Kellner L, Jahn C, Feichtinger H, Povelka M, Frohner U, Kruger A, Hilgers R-D et al (2002) Transplantation of autologous retinal pigment epithelium in eyes with foveal neovascularization resulting from age-related macular degeneration: a pilot study. Am J Ophthalmol 133:215–225

Del Priore LV, Kaplan HJ, Tezel TH, Hayashi N, Berger AS, Green WR (2001) Retinal pigment epithelial cell transplantation after subfoveal membranectomy in age-related macular degeneration: clinicopathologic correlation. Am J Ophthalmol 131:472–480

Drukker M, Katchman H, Katz G, Even-Tov Friedman S, Shezen E, Hornstein E, Mandelboim O, Reisner Y, Benvenisty N (2006) Human embryonic stem cells and their differentiated derivatives are less susceptible to immune rejection than adult cells. Stem Cells 24:221–229

Flood MT, Gouras P, Kjeldbye H (1980) Growth characteristics and ultrastructure of human retinal pigment epithelium in vitro. Invest Ophthalmol Vis Sci 19:1309–1320

Gal A, Li Y, Thompson DA, Weir J, Orth U, Jacobson SG, Apfelstedt-Sylla E, Vollrath D (2000) Mutations in MERTK, the human orthologue of the RCS rat retinal dystrophy gene, cause retinitis pigmentosa. Nat Genet 26:270–271

Gouras P, Flood MT, Kjeldbye H (1984) Transplantation of cultured human retinal cells to monkey retina. An Acad Bras Cienc 56:431–443

Gouras P, Flood MT, Kjeldbye H, Bilek MK, Eggers H (1985) Transplantation of cultured human retinal epithelium to Bruch's membrane of the owl monkey's eye. Curr Eye Res 4:253–265

Klimanskaya I, Hipp J, Rezai KA, West M, Atala A, Lanza R (2004) Derivation and comparative assessment of retinal pigment epithelium from human embryonic stem cells using transcriptomics. Cloning Stem Cells 6:217–245

Koenekoop RK (2003) The gene for Stargardt disease, ABCA4, is a major retinal gene: a mini-review. Ophthalmic Genet 24:75–80

Koenekoop RK, Lopez I, den Hollander AI, Allikmets R, Cremers FPM (2007) Genetic testing for retinal dystrophies and dysfunctions: benefits, dilemmas and solutions. Clin Experiment Ophthalmol 35: 473–485

Lopez R, Gouras P, Kjeldbye H, Sullivan B, Reppucci V, Brittis M, Wapner F, Goluboff E (1989) Transplanted retinal pigment epithelium modifies the retinal degeneration in the RCS rat. Invest Ophthalmol Vis Sci 30:586–588

Lu B, Malcuit C, Wang S, Girman S, Francis P, Lemieux L, Lanza R, Lund R (2009) Long-term safety and function of RPE from human embryonic stem cells in preclinical models of macular degeneration. Stem Cells 27:2126–2135

Lund RD, Wang S, Klimanskaya I, Holmes T, Ramos-Kelsey R, Lu B, Girman S, Bischoff N, Sauve Y, Lanza R (2006) Human embryonic stem cell-derived cells rescue visual function in dystrophic RCS rats. Cloning Stem Cells 8:189–199

Lund RD, Wang S, Lu B, Girman S, Holmes T, Sauve Y, Messina DJ, Harris IR, Kihm AJ, Harmon AM et al (2007) Cells isolated from umbilical cord tissue rescue photoreceptors and visual functions in a rodent model of retinal disease. Stem Cells 25:602–611

Okamura RM, Lebkowski J, Au M, Priest CA, Denham J, Majumdar AS (2007) Immunological properties of human embryonic stem cell-derived oligodendrocyte progenitor cells. J Neuroimmunol 192:134–144

Pan CK, Heilweil G, Lanza R, Schwartz SD (2013) Embryonic stem cells as a treatment for macular degeneration. Expert Opin Biol Ther 13:1125–1133

Peyman GA, Blinder KJ, Paris CL, Alturki W, Nelson NC Jr, Desai U (1991) A technique for retinal pigment epithelium transplantation for age-related macular degeneration secondary to extensive subfoveal scarring. Ophthalmic Surg 22:102–108

Schwartz SD, Hubschman J-P, Heilwell G, Franco-Cardenas V, Pan CK, Ostrick RM, Mickunas E, Gay R, Klimanskaya I, Lanza R (2012) Embryonic stem cell trials for macular degeneration: a preliminary report. Lancet 379(9817):713–720

Sun H, Nathans J (1997) Stargardt's ABCR is localized to the disc membrane of retinal rod outer segments. Nat Genet 17:15–16

Travis GH, Golczak M, Moise AR, Palczewski K (2007) Diseases caused by defects in the visual cycle: retinoids as potential therapeutic agents. Annu Rev Pharmacol Toxicol 47:469–512

van Meurs JC, ter Averst E, Hofland LJ, van Hagen PM, Mooy CM, Baarsma GS, Kuijpers RW, Boks T, Stalmans P (2004) Autologous peripheral retinal pigment epithelium translocation in patients with subfoveal neovascular membranes. Br J Ophthalmol 88:110–113

Weng J, Mata NL, Azarian SM, Tzekov RT, Birch DG, Travis GH (1999) Insights into the function of Rim protein in photoreceptors and etiology of Stargardt's disease from the phenotype in abcr knockout mice. Cell 98:13–23

Wenkel H, Streilein JW (1998) Analysis of immune deviation elicited by antigens injected into the subretinal space. Invest Ophthalmol Vis Sci 39:1823–1834

Restoring Physiologic Barriers Against Neovascular Invasion

Cecinio C. Ronquillo Jr., Samuel F. Passi, and Balamurali K. Ambati

8.1 The Road to Treat ARMD

Age-related macular degeneration is a complex disease. In complex problems, several perspectives are needed to understand basic mechanisms underlying disease pathophysiology. Our perspective of ARMD as a neovascular disease stems from our early studies on corneal neovascularization (Ambati et al. 2002). In a chemically induced mouse corneal neovascularization model, we showed the first evidence of using a biological molecule for preventing corneal neovascularization. Since then, we found other molecules important for inhibiting corneal neovascularization in a nonphysiological system (Ambati et al. 2003a, b; Sakurai et al. 2003). At that point, the physiological mechanism of maintaining corneal avascularity was still not known. The dogma then was that

multiple redundant pathways controlled avascularity in the cornea.

In 2006, we reported that expression of soluble VEGF receptor-1 (sFLT-1) is necessary and sufficient for maintenance of corneal avascularity (Ambati et al. 2006). Moreover, we showed that the mechanism of sFLT-1 was through sequestration of VEGF-A leading to inhibition of function. In the next few years, we showed that this same pathway was responsible for maintaining the avascular photoreceptor layer of the retina (Luo et al. 2013a). In ARMD, the avascular photoreceptor layer is penetrated by blood vessels, leading to choroidal neovascularization (CNV). This loss of barrier function of the photoreceptor layer may be due in part to loss of sFLT-1 leading to VEGF-A-induced neovascularization.

As sFlt-1 became a clinically attractive platform for inhibiting VEGF-A for several neovascular diseases including ARMD (Lukason et al. 2011; Lai et al. 2012), we continued to search for other strategies for VEGF-A inhibition. Most of the strategies for VEGF-A inhibition including sFlt-1 focused on inhibiting VEGF-A after it is secreted from the cell; however, it has been shown that VEGF can act via an intracellular autocrine loop which is currently not being targeted by current approaches (Gerber et al. 2002). We then began formulating strategies to inhibit VEGF-A intracellularly before the protein can be secreted from the cell. Although the implication of autocrine signaling in the context of neovascularization is unclear, addition of strategies inhibiting this

C.C. Ronquillo Jr., PhD • S.F. Passi, BA
Department of Ophthalmology and Visual Sciences, John A. Moran Eye Center, University of Utah Health Sciences Center, University of Utah School of Medicine, Salt Lake City, UT, USA
e-mail: nikko.ronquillo@hsc.utah.edu; samuel.passi@hsc.utah.edu

B.K. Ambati, MD, PhD, MBA (⌗)
Department of Ophthalmology and Visual Sciences, John A. Moran Eye Center, University of Utah Health Sciences Center, University of Utah School of Medicine, Salt Lake City, UT, USA

Department of Ophthalmology, University of Utah, Salt Lake City, UT, USA
e-mail: bala.ambati@utah.edu

E.P. Rakoczy (ed.), *Gene- and Cell-Based Treatment Strategies for the Eye*, Essentials in Ophthalmology, DOI 10.1007/978-3-662-45188-5_8, © Springer-Verlag Berlin Heidelberg 2015 pathway may result in better control of disease, because if vascular endothelial cells express their own growth factors and receptors, extracellular blockade alone may be insufficient.

8.2   Identification of the Gene

Flt-1 (fms-like tyrosine kinase-1) is a transmembrane receptor in the tyrosine kinase family that was first identified in a v-ros oncogene hybridization screen (Shibuya et al. 1990). A couple of years after its identification, it was found that Flt-1 was a high-affinity receptor for VEGF (de Vries et al. 1992).

The 180 kDa Flt-1 protein is known to have seven immunoglobulin (Ig)-like domains in the extracellular region and a tyrosine kinase domain (Shibuya et al. 1990). The extracellular domain is important for ligand binding. Targeted mutation of mouse flt-1 resulted in a disorganized vasculature with embryonic lethality in homozygous animals (Fong et al. 1995). However, deleting only the tyrosine kinase domain was able to produce viable mice that developed normal blood vessels (Hiratsuka et al. 1998). These studies suggested that the ligand-binding domain of Flt-1 was necessary for normal angiogenesis.

The ligand for Flt-1 is VEGF with binding constants in the picomolar range (Davis-Smyth et al. 1996). Crystallographic studies on VEGF-Flt-1 interaction showed that the second and third extracellular domains of Flt-1 are necessary and sufficient for binding VEGF at close to the native binding affinities (Wiesmann et al. 1997).

Since the initial discovery of Flt-1, many studies have looked into the mechanism for VEGF signaling in vivo. Its strong binding affinity with VEGF has enabled us to use Flt-1 as a biological "bait" to sequester VEGF.

8.3   Identification of the Delivery Vector

The current approved treatment for the neovascularization in ARMD is injection of VEGF inhibitors to the vitreous. One limitation for this strategy is the need for recurrent injections (once every 4–6 weeks) into the eye of patients to maintain active VEGF suppression. Current research in this area focuses on (a) developing longer-term strategies for inhibition of VEGF and (b) efficient therapeutic delivery to the eye without the need for direct intravitreal injections (e.g., intravenous-based therapies, oral therapies).

Gene therapy-based strategies are effective for longer-term expression of VEGF inhibitors. Two mechanisms currently exist for gene delivery: using viral vectors (e.g., adeno-associated virus or AAV) and nonviral systems. Several groups are developing AAV-based vectors for delivery of sFlt-1 (soluble Flt-1 receptor) to inhibit VEGF (Lai et al. 2012; Lukason et al. 2011). These studies have shown long-term inhibition of neovascularization after a single subretinal or intravitreal injection of AAV-sFlt in nonhuman primate models of choroidal neovascularization. One disadvantage for using viral vectors is still the need for invasive subretinal or intravitreal injections.

We adopted a nonviral system for Flt-1 delivery to the eye. Specifically, we used poly(lactic-co-glycolic acid) (PLGA) nanoparticles because of its several properties including (a) biodegradability and biocompatibility, (b) possibility to functionalize the nanoparticle to increase target cell specificity, (c) protection of cargo from degradation before reaching the target, and (d) PLGA nanoparticles that are already FDA approved for parenteral administration as drug delivery vehicles (Danhier et al. 2012).

To add target specificity of the PLGA nanoparticles and enhance delivery of its cargo to certain cells, we functionalized the surface of these nanoparticles with a peptide sequence containing the RGD motif (arginine-glycine-aspartic acid) (Singh et al. 2009). It is known that the peptide GRGDSPK binds integrin alpha v beta-3 receptors, which are commonly overexpressed in the blood vessels of patients with ARMD or diabetic retinopathy (Friedlander et al. 1996). We were able to show that intravenous administration of RGD-tagged PLGA nanoparticles containing Flt-1 was able to localize specifically to the neovascular eye of a rat CNV model and inhibit progression of CNV (Singh et al. 2009). We extended our studies to other neovascularization models in murine and nonhuman primates and showed similar results (see below) (Luo et al. 2013b).

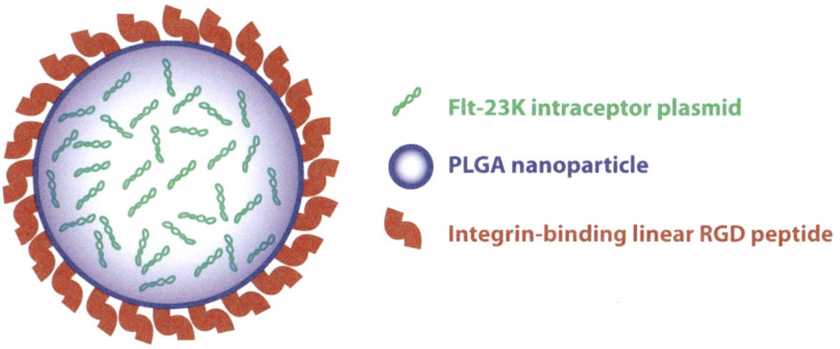

Fig. 8.1 Schematic representation of Flt23K plasmid loaded in PLGA nanoparticles. The surface of nanoparticles has been conjugated with the peptide, RGD, which increases specificity of the vector to target areas of neovascularization (Reprinted with permission from Luo et al. (2013a, b). Copyright 2013 American Chemical Society)

8.4 The Construct

Inhibiting VEGF intracellularly necessitates at least two prerequisites: (a) finding a molecule that binds VEGF at high affinity and (b) a molecule that has to be located intracellularly. The VEGF receptor-1 or VEGFR-1/Flt-1 was a good candidate because of its high binding affinity to VEGF. However, Flt-1 is normally secreted from the cell. Therefore, we needed a strategy to keep Flt-1 inside the to bind and sequester VEGF.

Flt-1 is known to have seven domains. Of these, the first domain contained the secretion signal sequence, the second and third domains are known to bind VEGF in nearly wild-type affinity compared to the intact protein, and the fourth domain is also thought to help in VEGF binding. To prevent Flt-1 from being secreted, we made an N-terminal truncation mutation, removing domain 1. Additionally, we engineered the truncated Flt-1 to contain a C-terminal KDEL tag (Singh et al. 2005). The KDEL tag is a peptide sequence (Lys-Asp-Glu-Leu) that binds endoplasmic reticulum receptors, preventing proteins containing this tag from being secreted (Lewis and Pelham 1990).

We initially tested two different constructs, Flt23K (Flt-1 domains 2 and 3 with KDEL tag) and Flt24K (Flt-1 domains 2, 3, and 4 with KDEL tag), for VEGF inhibition in vitro (Singh et al. 2005).

8.5 In Vitro Data

We used a human cornea epithelial cell culture model to determine whether KDEL-tagged Flt23K and Flt24K are able to inhibit VEGF secretion. In this model, we are able to upregulate expression of VEGF by placing the cells in a hypoxic environment. Both constructs were able to remain intracellularly, in close association with the endoplasmic reticulum. After overexpression of Flt23K or Flt24K, we showed that compared to Flt24K and control cell lines, Flt23K is able to significantly reduce VEGF secretion from the cells. These results were promising, and we tested whether KDEL-tagged Flt23K is able to inhibit neovascularization in in vivo animal models. We used the PLGA nanoparticles as vectors for Flt23K.

8.6 The Tests and Results

Our overall strategy for VEGF inhibition in vivo used the Flt23K intraceptor loaded in RGD-functionalized PLGA nanoparticles (Fig. 8.1). First, we explored whether RGD-functionalized PLGA nanoparticles can specifically localize to CNV lesions with intravenous loading. Using a laser-induced CNV mouse model with one eye laser treated and the other eye as the control, we intravenously administered nanoparticles labeled with the Nile Red tracer with or without RGD. We showed that nanoparticles can specifically localize to the laser-treated eye but not to the control eye (Fig. 8.2).

We then proceeded to investigate whether active targeting of our nanoparticles by surface functionalization with RGD could enhance nanoparticle localization and ultimately gene delivery to CNV lesions. Using confocal microscopy, we were able to compare relative

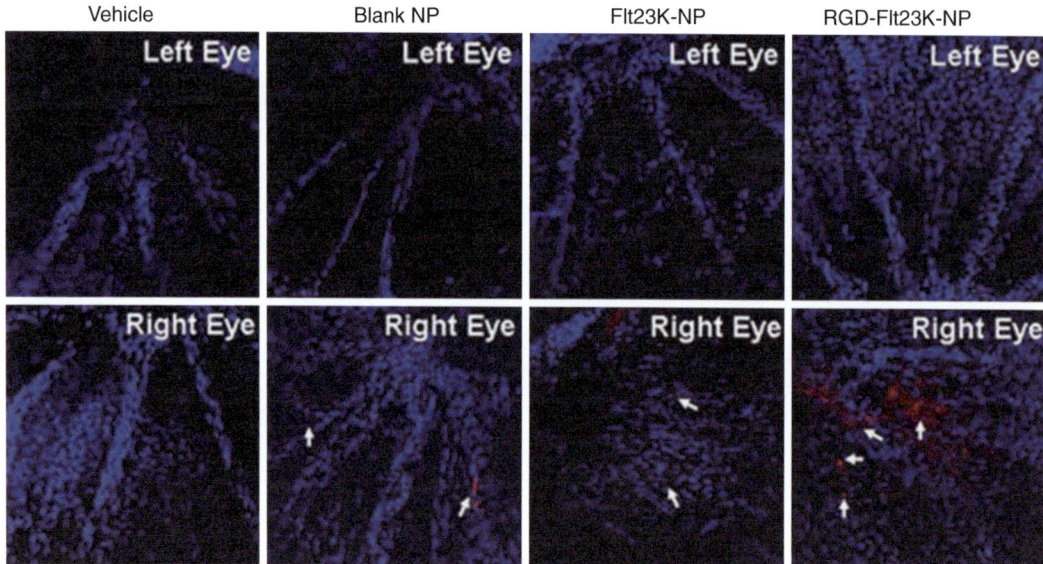

Fig. 8.2 Intravenously administered RGD-functionalized nanoparticles are specifically delivered to laser-treated rat eyes. Nanoparticles were injected into the tail veins of Brown Norway (BN) rats 14 days after laser treatment of the right eye. Eyes were harvested 24 h after nanoparticle injection. Representative flatmounts of laser-treated right eyes (*bottom row*) and control left eyes (*top row*) were imaged by confocal microscopy. Nanoparticles alone or nanoparticles loaded with the Flt23K plasmid showed minimal targeting to laser-treated eyes. However, nanoparticles functionalized with the RGD peptide loaded with Flt23K plasmid showed increased targeting to laser-treated eyes. Nanoparticles (*red, nile red* (*white arrows*)), DAPI (*blue*) (Reproduced and modified from Singh et al. (2009))

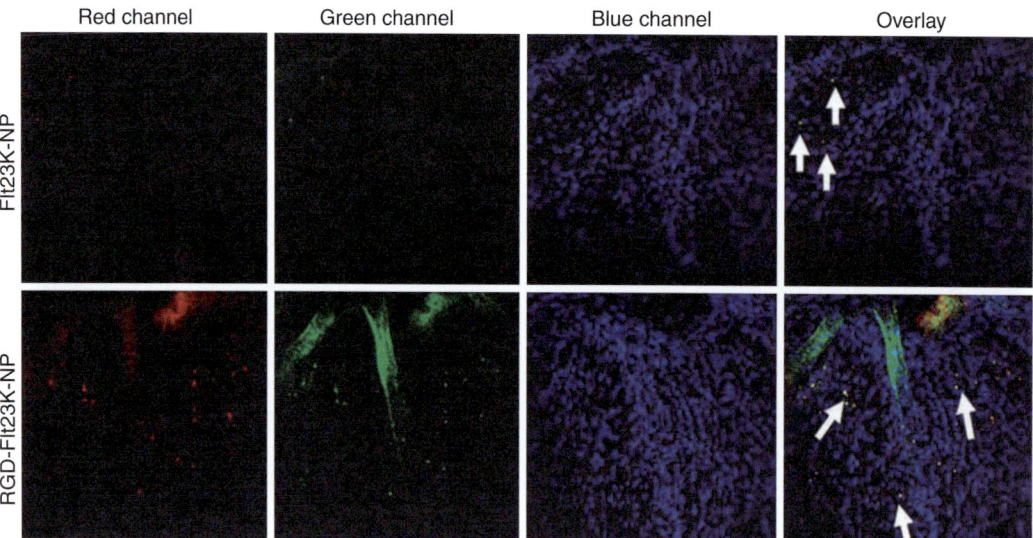

Fig. 8.3 Flt23K expression in laser-treated rat eyes. Nanoparticles were injected into the tail veins of Brown Norway (BN) rats 14 days after laser treatment of the right eye. Eyes were harvested 24 h after nanoparticle injection. Representative flatmounts of laser-treated right eyes injected with unconjugated Flt23K-plasmid-loaded nanoparticles (Flt23K-NP) and RGD-peptide-conjugated Flt23K-plasmid-loaded nanoparticles (RGD-Flt23K-NP). Only the RGD-conjugated nanoparticles showed increased expression of Flt23K in the laser-treated eyes. Flt23K (*green*, GFP), nanoparticles (*red, nile red* (*white arrows*)), DAPI (*blue*) (Reproduced and modified from Singh et al. (2009))

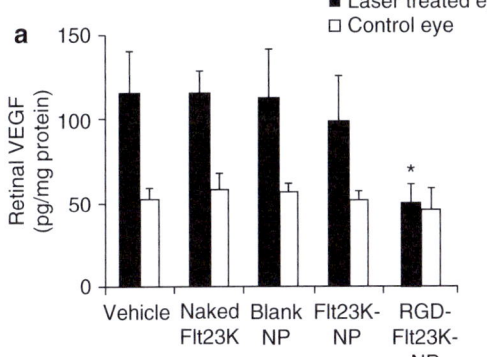

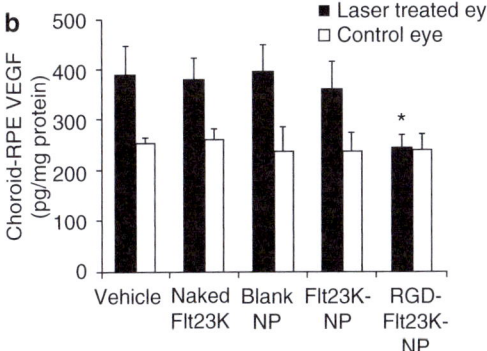

Fig. 8.4 Functionalized nanoparticles reduce (**a**) retinal and (**b**) choroidal-RPE vascular endothelial growth factor (VEGF) levels. On day 14 after choroidal neovascularization (CNV) induction, the rats were administered one of the following treatments by injection into the tail vein: (1) vehicle, (2) naked Flt23K plasmid, (3) blank nanoparticles, (4) unconjugated Flt23K-plasmid-loaded nanoparticles (Flt23K-NP), and (5) RGD-peptide-conjugated Flt23K-plasmid-loaded nanoparticles (RGD-Flt23K-NP). The rats were euthanized 48 h after nanoparticle injection. Neural retina and choroid-RPE were dissected, and VEGF levels were quantified by sandwich enzyme-linked immunosorbent assay (ELISA). *$P < 0.05$ as compared to vehicle, naked Flt23K, blank nanoparticles, and nonfunctionalized nanoparticle-treated groups (Reproduced and modified from Singh et al. (2009))

concentrations of Nile Red-labeled nanoparticles and green fluorescent protein-labeled Flt23K intraceptor, of both nonfunctionalized and functionalized nanoparticles. Our results show that functionalized nanoparticles increased localization and Flt23K expression to CNV lesions compared to nanoparticles that did not have RGD functionalization (Fig. 8.3).

Next, we assessed whether functionalized nanoparticles loaded with Flt23K were capable of reducing retinal and choroidal-RPE levels of VEGF in the laser-treated, neovascular eye. At baseline, laser-treated eyes had markedly elevated VEGF levels when compared to control eyes as was expected. Targeted expression of Flt23K inhibited VEGF levels down to baseline levels comparable with the control eye (Fig. 8.4).

Finally, we wanted to test whether Flt23K-loaded nanoparticles are able to inhibit CNV. Using both histopathologic examination and FITC-dextran analysis of choroidal flat-mounts, we were able to quantify the areas of CNV lesions in each eye. We observed a significant reduction in the area of CNV lesions in the laser-treated eyes treated with functionalized nanoparticles delivering Flt23K. These results suggest a possible therapeutic role for Flt23K loaded in RGD-functionalized PLGA nanoparticles in the treatment of neovascular or wet ARMD (Fig. 8.5).

Having refined our method of Flt23K intraceptor delivery and expression utilizing functionalized nanoparticles and showing efficacy at inhibiting laser-induced CNV, we further explored its potential therapeutic benefits in both a mouse and primate ARMD model. Specifically, we were interested in defining the role of our gene therapy strategy on (a) angiogenesis and fibrosis, (b) its safety profile, and (c) exploring its therapeutic potential in restoring visual loss induced by CNV.

Current intravitreal injection protein-based therapies, although successful at reducing CNV-associated angiogenesis, are limited by their inability to address the concomitant fibrosis, which often accompanies CNV in the pathogenesis of ARMD. Thus, in addition to confirming the ability of our particle to inhibit angiogenesis, we wanted to investigate its ability to inhibit fibrosis. Just as we had previously shown in rat, we were able to demonstrate that targeted expression of Flt23K using nanoparticles as a vector was able to reduce angiogenesis in murine and primate laser-induced models as evidenced by decreasing CNV surface volumes (Fig. 8.6).

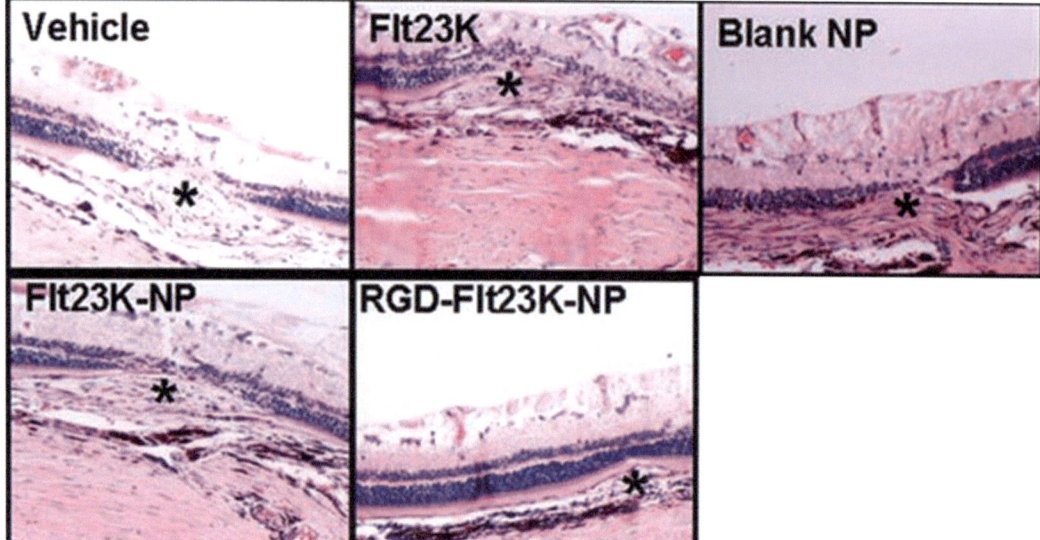

Fig. 8.5 Functionalized nanoparticles reduce laser-induced choroidal neovascular area on histopathologic examination. On day 14 after choroidal neovascularization (CNV) induction, the rats were administered one of the following treatments intravenously: (1) vehicle, (2) naked Flt23K plasmid, (3) blank nanoparticles, (4) unconjugated Flt23K-plasmid-loaded nanoparticles (Flt23K-NP), and (5) RGD-peptide-conjugated Flt23K-plasmid-loaded nanoparticles (RGD-Flt23K-NP). The rats were euthanized 2 weeks after nanoparticle injection. Only the RGD-Flt23K-NP group was able to decrease CNV area significantly. *Astricks* represents CNV lesions (Reproduced and modified from Singh et al. (2009))

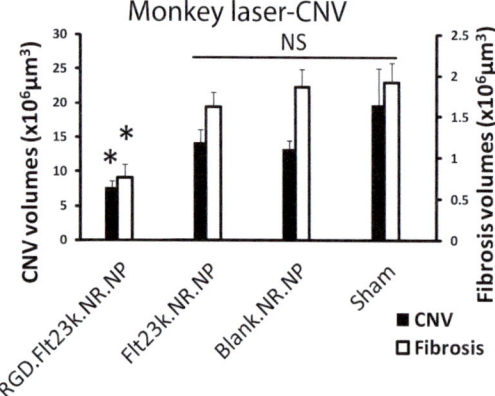

Fig. 8.6 RGD-functionalized nanoparticles loaded with Flt23K inhibit CNV and fibrosis. In the laser-induced CNV monkey model, the volumes of CNV lesions (*asterisk*), including neovessels (stained by perlecan) and fibrosis (stained by collagen I), significantly decreased 4 weeks after RGD.Flt23k.NR.NP treatment. (Reprinted with permission from Luo et al. (2013a, b). Copyright 2013 American Chemical Society)

We also showed that this strategy was able to significantly reduce fibrosis in the same model (Fig. 8.6).

Although inhibition of CNV is important for decreasing disease burden, functional restoration of visual function is the ultimate goal for patients with ARMD. Unfortunately, with current intravitreal therapy, many patients do not achieve substantial visual improvement, and up to a third of treated eyes progress to legal blindness (Rofagha et al. 2013). While laser-induced CNV models are widely used to study ARMD, they are limited due to the laser's acute injury and retinal burnout, which results in no potential for recovery of visual function. Consequently, to investigate the role of Flt23K on visual restoration, we created a novel mouse model of ARMD. We induced neovascularization in a mouse by targeting AAV particles containing sFlt-1 shRNA to the retina.

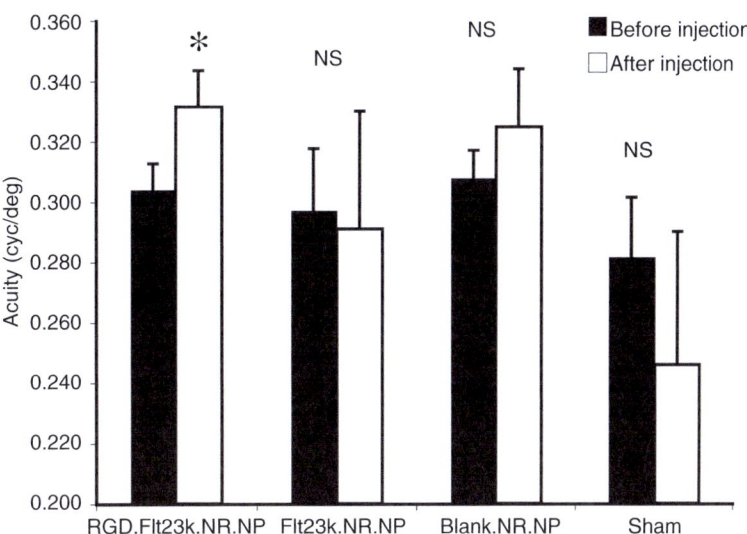

Fig. 8.7 RGD-functionalized nanoparticles loaded with Flt23K improve vision. Optomotor tested vision function was partially restored after 4-week treatment with RGD.Flt23k.NR.NP but not with the vehicle or sham controls. *Astricks* represents CNV lesions (Reprinted with permission from Luo et al. (2013a, b). Copyright 2013 American Chemical Society)

By administering a subretinal injection of adeno-associated viral (AAV)-short hairpin RNA (shRNA) targeted against sFlt-1 (a naturally occurring inhibitor of VEGF inhibitor), we were able to create a reversible model of CNV with which we could test nanoparticle-delivered Flt23K. Following intravenous injection of nanoparticles loaded with Flt23K, we were able to observe progressive visual acuity improvement of greater than 10 % in the eyes of the treatment group (Fig. 8.7).

Lastly, we sought to define the safety profile of RGD.Flt23k.NR.NP. Analyzing the serum 1 day post IV administration, no quantifiable Nile Red was identified, suggesting the amounts of nanoparticles remaining in the bloodstream 24 h after injection was negligible. Additionally, at 30 days postinjection, although present in CNV lesions, no quantifiable amount of Nile Red was found in extraocular tissues including the kidney, lung, liver, and skin. Fundoscopic exam was also performed to assess for the presence of ocular toxicity, and the results showed no evidence of hemorrhage, inflation, retinal detachment, or retinal degeneration. H&E staining also failed to demonstrate any retinal morphologic abnormalities.

Finally, using TUNEL staining, we demonstrated the absence of retinal apoptosis outside the area of CNV lesions.

Inspired by the current limitations of intravitreal injections in anti-VEGF therapy, we showed that nanoparticle-mediated delivery of Flt23K is able to inhibit ARMD-associated fibrosis and effectively restore CNV-associated vision loss while simultaneously maintaining a reassuring systemic and ocular safety profile.

8.7 Future Plans

Our recent studies have shown that intravenous injection of Flt23K loaded in surface-functionalized nanoparticles in rat, murine, and primate models of CNV is able to significantly suppress choroidal neovascularization. We have also shown that this strategy is also effective in inhibition of fibrosis. Inhibition of fibrosis is an important clinical problem that is not currently addressed by current therapies. Although the mechanism is unclear, it is likely that suppression of fibrosis is through RGD-mediated inhibition of collagen production as previously reported

(Kotoh et al. 2004). Moreover, nanoparticle-based delivery of Flt23K in primates did not show any obvious acute toxicity issues. More studies need to be conducted to assess long-term toxicity issues.

As PLGA nanoparticles are already FDA approved as a nonviral drug delivery vector, it is our vision to conduct a Phase I clinical trial on the safety of RGD-functionalized nanoparticles loaded with Flt23K in humans. Our long-term vision for this strategy is to test whether it is sufficient to inhibit progression or regress neovascularization in CNV and other pathologies including corneal neovascularization either as monotherapy or as an adjunct to current anti-VEGF therapies.

Compliance with Ethical Requirements

Conflict of Interest Author Balamurali K. Ambati declares that he has issued a patent on the technologies discussed in the chapter.

Author Samuel F. Passi declares that he has no conflict of interest.

Author Cecinio C. Ronquillo declares that he has no conflict of interest.

Informed Consent All procedures followed were in accordance with the ethical standards of the responsible committee on human experimentation (institutional and national) and with the Helsinki Declaration of 1975, as revised in 2000. Informed consent was obtained from all patients for being included in the study.

Animal Studies All institutional and national guidelines for the care and use of laboratory animals were followed. All experiments were approved by the IACUCs of Medical College of Georgia, University of Colorado Denver, and University of Utah for the experiments performed at the respective sites.

References

Ambati BK, Joussen AM, Ambati J, Moromizato Y, Guha C, Javaherian K, Gillies S, O'Reilly MS, Adamis AP (2002) Angiostatin inhibits and regresses corneal neovascularization. Arch Ophthalmol 120(8): 1063–1068

Ambati BK, Anand A, Joussen AM, Kuziel WA, Adamis AP, Ambati J (2003a) Sustained inhibition of corneal neovascularization by genetic ablation of CCR5. Invest Ophthalmol Vis Sci 44(2):590–593

Ambati BK, Joussen AM, Kuziel WA, Adamis AP, Ambati J (2003b) Inhibition of corneal neovascularization by genetic ablation of CCR2. Cornea 22(5):465–467

Ambati BK, Nozaki M, Singh N, Takeda A, Jani PD, Suthar T, Albuquerque RJ, Richter E, Sakurai E, Newcomb MT, Kleinman ME, Caldwell RB, Lin Q, Ogura Y, Orecchia A, Samuelson DA, Agnew DW, St Leger J, Green WR, Mahasreshti PJ, Curiel DT, Kwan D, Marsh H, Ikeda S, Leiper LJ, Collinson JM, Bogdanovich S, Khurana TS, Shibuya M, Baldwin ME, Ferrara N, Gerber HP, De Falco S, Witta J, Baffi JZ, Raisler BJ, Ambati J (2006) Corneal avascularity is due to soluble VEGF receptor-1. Nature 443(7114):993–997

Danhier F, Ansorena E, Silva JM, Coco R, Le Breton A, Préat V (2012) PLGA-based nanoparticles: an overview of biomedical applications. J Control Release 161(2):505–522

Davis-Smyth T, Chen H, Park J, Presta LG, Ferrara N (1996) The second immunoglobulin-like domain of the VEGF tyrosine kinase receptor Flt-1 determines ligand binding and may initiate a signal transduction cascade. EMBO J 15(18):4919–4927

de Vries C, Escobedo JA, Ueno H, Houck K, Ferrara N, Williams LT (1992) The fms-like tyrosine kinase, a receptor for vascular endothelial growth factor. Science 255(5047):989–991

Fong GH, Rossant J, Gertsenstein M, Breitman ML (1995) Role of the Flt-1 receptor tyrosine kinase in regulating the assembly of vascular endothelium. Nature 376(6535):66–70

Friedlander M, Theesfeld CL, Sugita M, Fruttiger M, Thomas MA, Chang S, Cheresh DA (1996) Involvement of integrins alpha v beta 3 and alpha v beta 5 in ocular neovascular diseases. Proc Natl Acad Sci U S A 93(18):9764–9769

Gerber HP, Malik AK, Solar GP, Sherman D, Liang XH, Meng G, Hong K, Marsters JC, Ferrara N (2002) VEGF regulates haematopoietic stem cell survival by an internal autocrine loop mechanism. Nature 417(6892):954–958

Hiratsuka S, Minowa O, Kuno J, Noda T, Shibuya M (1998) Flt-1 lacking the tyrosine kinase domain is sufficient for normal development and angiogenesis in mice. Proc Natl Acad Sci U S A 95(16):9349–9354

Kotoh K, Nakamuta M, Kohjima M, Fukushima M, Morizono S, Kobayashi N, Enjoji M, Nawata H (2004) Arg-Gly-Asp (RGD) peptide ameliorates carbon tetrachloride-induced liver fibrosis via inhibition of collagen production and acceleration of collagenase activity. Int J Mol Med 14(6):1049–1053

Lai CM, Estcourt MJ, Himbeck RP, Lee SY, Yew-San Yeo I, Luu C, Loh BK, Lee MW, Barathi A, Villano J, Ang CL, van der Most RG, Constable IJ, Dismuke D, Samulski RJ, Degli-Esposti MA, Rakoczy EP (2012) Preclinical safety evaluation of subretinal AAV2.sFlt-1 in non-human primates. Gene Ther 19(10):999–1009

Lewis MJ, Pelham HR (1990) A human homologue of the yeast HDEL receptor. Nature 348(6297):162–163

Lukason M, DuFresne E, Rubin H, Pechan P, Li Q, Kim I, Kiss S, Flaxel C, Collins M, Miller J, Hauswirth W, Maclachlan T, Wadsworth S, Scaria A (2011) Inhibition of choroidal neovascularization in a nonhuman primate model by intravitreal administration of an AAV2 vector expressing a novel anti-VEGF molecule. Mol Ther 19(2):260–265

Luo L, Uehara H, Zhang X, Das SK, Olsen T, Holt D, Simonis JM, Jackman K, Singh N, Miya TR, Huang W, Ahmed F, Bastos-Carvalho A, Le YZ, Mamalis C, Chiodo VA, Hauswirth WW, Baffi J, Lacal PM, Orecchia A, Ferrara N, Gao G, Young-Hee K, Fu Y, Owen L, Albuquerque R, Baehr W, Thomas K, Li DY, Chalam KV, Shibuya M, Grisanti S, Wilson DJ, Ambati J, Ambati BK (2013a) Photoreceptor avascular privilege is shielded by soluble VEGF receptor-1. Elife 2:e00324. doi:10.7554/eLife.00324

Luo L, Zhang X, Hirano Y, Tyagi P, Barabás P, Uehara H, Miya TR, Singh N, Archer B, Qazi Y, Jackman K, Das SK, Olsen T, Chennamaneni SR, Stagg BC, Ahmed F, Emerson L, Zygmunt K, Whitaker R, Mamalis C, Huang W, Gao G, Srinivas SP, Krizaj D, Baffi J, Ambati J, Kompella UB, Ambati BK (2013b) Targeted intraceptor nanoparticle therapy reduces angiogenesis and fibrosis in primate and murine macular degeneration. ACS Nano 7(4):3264–3275

Rofagha S, Bhisitkul RB, Boyer DS, Sadda SR, Zhang K, SEVEN-UP Study Group (2013) Seven-year outcomes in ranibizumab-treated patients in ANCHOR, MARINA, and HORIZON: a multicenter

cohort study (SEVEN-UP). Ophthalmology 120(11): 2292–2299

Sakurai E, Taguchi H, Anand A, Ambati BK, Gragoudas ES, Miller JW, Adamis AP, Ambati J (2003) Targeted disruption of the CD18 or ICAM-1 gene inhibits choroidal neovascularization. Invest Ophthalmol Vis Sci 44(6):2743–2749

Shibuya M, Yamaguchi S, Yamane A, Ikeda T, Tojo A, Matsushime H, Sato M (1990) Nucleotide sequence and expression of a novel human receptor-type tyrosine kinase gene (flt) closely related to the fms family. Oncogene 5(4):519–524

Singh N, Amin S, Richter E, Rashid S, Scoglietti V, Jani PD, Wang J, Kaur R, Ambati J, Dong Z, Ambati BK (2005) Flt-1 intraceptors inhibit hypoxia-induced VEGF expression in vitro and corneal neovascularization in vivo. Invest Ophthalmol Vis Sci 46(5):1647–1652

Singh SR, Grossniklaus HE, Kang SJ, Edelhauser HF, Ambati BK, Kompella UB (2009) Intravenous transferrin, RGD peptide and dual-targeted nanoparticles enhance anti-VEGF intraceptor gene delivery to laser-induced CNV. Gene Ther 16(5):645–659

Wiesmann C, Fuh G, Christinger HW, Eigenbrot C, Wells JA, De Vos AM (1997) Crystal structure at 1.7 A resolution of VEGF in complex with domain 2 of the Flt-1 receptor. Cell 91(5):695–704